CARING: THE COMPASSION AND WISDOM OF NURSING

CARING: THE COMPASSION AND WISDOM OF NURSING

Edited by

Gosia Brykczyńska BA, BSc, Dip PH, Cert Ed,
RGN, RSCN, ONC Cert

Lecturer in Ethics and Philosophy
Royal College of Nursing Institute
London, UK

Editorial Adviser

Moya Jolley MA (Ed), BSc (Econ), SRN, Dip Ed,
RNT, Dip in Nursing (London)

Former Lecturer in Sociology and Nursing Development
Royal College of Nursing Institute
London, UK

SINGULAR PUBLISHING GROUP, INC.
San Diego, California

First published in Great Britain in 1997

© 1997 Arnold

Published and distributed in the United States and Canada by
SINGULAR PUBLISHING GROUP, Inc. 401 West "A" Street, Suite 325,
San Diego, California 92101-7904, USA

Whilst the advice and information in this book is believed to be true and
accurate at the date of going to press, neither the authors nor the publisher
can accept any legal responsibility or liability for any errors or omissions
that may be made. In particular (but without limiting the generality of the
preceding disclaimer) every effort has been made to check drug dosages;
however it is still possible that errors have been missed. Furthermore,
dosage schedules are constantly being revised and new side-effects
recognized. For these reasons the reader is strongly urged to consult the
drug companies' printed instructions before administering any of the drugs
recommended in this book.

Library of Congress Cataloging-in-Publication Data
A catalog record for this book is available from the Library of Congress

ISBN 1-56593-769-4

Printed and bound in Great Britain

Contents

List of contributors

Dr Ann Bradshaw, PhD, Dip N, SRN
Macmillan Lecturer in Palliative Nursing, RCN Institute, Oxford, UK

Ms Gosia Brykczyńska, BA, BSc, Dip PH, Cert Ed, RGN, RSCN, RNT
Lecturer in Ethics and Philosophy, Royal College of Nursing, London, UK

Dr Philip Burnard, PhD, MSc, RGN, RMN, Dip N, Cert Ed, RNT
Reader in Nursing Studies, University of Wales College of Medicine, Cardiff, UK

Dr Carol Cox, PhD, MSc, MA, PGDip Ed, BSc, RN
Head of the Department of Nursing, St Bartholomew School of Nursing, City University, London, UK

Dr Meg McDonald, PhD, BA, RGN, DN, CPT
Practice Nurse, East London, UK

Dr Paul Morrison, PhD, BA, RMN, RGN, PGCE, C Psychol, AFBPsS
Associate Professor, School of Nursing, Faculty of Health, Queensland University of Technology, Brisbane, Australia

Dr Pam Smith, PhD, MSc, B Nurs
Research Fellow, School of Health, University of Greenwich, London, UK, and **Ms Ellen Agard**, RN, MPH
PhD Candidate, Graduate Theological Union, Berkeley, CA, USA

Ms Verena Tschudin, MSc, BSc(Hons), Dip Counselling, RGN, RMN
Senior Lecturer, University of East London, UK, and Editor, International Journal of *Nursing Ethics*

Preface

Most of the professional nursing literature on caring, caring theories and constructs of caring is North American in origin. Whereas geography alone does not determine the analysis of concepts of caring, it does affect availability and ease of access to the literature. The European nurse is not likely to locate the North American caring literature with ease in libraries or even in university bookshops. For this reason, the following collection of essays on various aspects of caring, written by nursing scholars and leaders, has been presented to the European nursing readership. It is aimed predominantly at qualified nurses and those studying for academic degrees in nursing and health-care studies.

This is a collection of essays which can be read as a whole, giving an academically sound overview of thoughts on caring as they are understood by leaders of the profession today. The collection can also be approached piecemeal, with the reader delving into specific chapters as and when he or she sees the need. No attempt has been made to standardize the styles of writing, intellectual perspectives or academic assumptions. There are many ways of approaching caring, and many definitions of what it means to care, to be cared for, to experience care, and to share caring. Therefore the far-ranging limits of caring are reflected in the authors' eclectic approach to the subject.

The areas covered range from a brief overview of caring theories to an historical appreciation of our European traditions of caring. This is followed by an appreciation of the ethical implications of caring in a profession where one has a duty to care and the spiritual dimensions of caring are all too often overlooked. A chapter on the interrelationship of the humanities with caring arts is contrasted with the fundamental *sine qua non*, that all caring needs to be manifested within a context of competency. Indeed it is because one is competent that one can be caring. There is a tendency in the caring literature to overlook the patient's experience of being cared for, and any research that illustrates patients' and clients' perceptions of being cared for is of immense value to this field of inquiry. The truism that we are people first and patients' second is often forgotten, or only marginally acknowledged. Before we ever seek professional caring intervention, however, we develop our own culturally supported caring rituals. In our multi-ethnic society we forget that not all people will have the same caring strategies, a point that is brought out by the chapter on caring rituals among Gujurati women. Caring in a professional sense cannot be seen in isolation from caring behaviours we engage in by ourselves at home. Professional caring, however, can cause us much angst and emotional struggle. As nurses promoting a caring approach to our work, how much time do we spend considering how to offset burn-out, prevent disillusionment, or analyse the stressful nature of caring? Finally, the last chapter acknowledges the realities of caring costs, the gender aspects of the caring profession and the wider implications of the political and social context within which we have to work as caring nurses, and it suggests a new way of looking at caring theories.

The opening essay draws attention to the professional paradox of caring. Caring is seen as the highly skilled art of nursing, and yet it is very ordinary in its necessity. The book closes with an essay commenting on the labour and cost of caring for a predominantly female work force, and suggests a theory of caring that needs to be explored further by the profession. Meanwhile, however one views caring, one thing is certain, that to care is human, and our professionalization of caring must never obscure the ordinariness and naturalness of this act. The task of the profession is to promote caring where it is flagging, and to encourage new ways of caring when old techniques are not working. Its onerous task is to appreciate the human value that caring signifies for us, and to acknowledge its 'humanizing' effects on us. Sister Simon Roach (1992) refers to the innate desire which humans have to demonstrate care. It is, she states, the human mode of being. If caring is seen as this human 'norm', let us start to promote this human mode of being, this nursing normality. The more we understand about caring, the better we shall be able to promote this ordinary yet ennobling and creative art. I trust that this collection of essays will help the reader to understand a little more about the human mode of being and nursing's caring norms.

Gosia Brykczyńska
London, 1996

Acknowledgements

No book is ever written in isolation or without much indebtedness to many other people. First, I would especially like to thank my colleagues who contributed essays to the book, and my students at the Institute of the Royal College of Nursing whom I have been privileged to know over the last few years. It was during sessions on moral philosophy and the humanities that it became increasingly clear that they would appreciate a book consisting of a collection of essays on the many varied aspects of caring. They have also always been supportive of many of my projects, and have been my best guide to both the academic level and appropriateness of the proposed material in the book.

I would also like to thank Sue Hinchliff for her many varied ways of demonstrating support, Elizabeth Hillman for her excellent administrative and typing help (without her the manuscript would never have been completed) and Maria Bniński for her administrative help and much needed moral support. Finally, I would like to thank both Richard Holloway and Fiona Goodgame of Edward Arnold for their constant help and trust in the outcome of the project. Last but not least, I would like to thank Moya Jolley, who has been not only a valuable adviser throughout this undertaking, but also a great role model and mentor – a truly wise and caring nurse.

Gosia Brykczyńska
London, 1996

1

A brief overview of the epistemology of caring

Gosia Brykczyńska

This short chapter provides an overview of caring theories, and is intended to provide for the reader with minimal previous exposure to caring theories a relatively brief comprehensive survey of the subject. Because of the centrality of caring in nursing practice, many nurse theorists have looked at and analysed caring constructs and caring concepts. This chapter is intended as an introduction to the many arguments and perspectives that surround these caring theories. Caring in nursing practice is a core concept, because it concerns a fundamental aspect of nursing. Without the presence of a wise, caring, compassionate approach to the delivery of nursing, the nursing tasks would be seen as faulted. Without caring, nursing would represent an incomplete or even disingenuous and non-efficacious picture of what it is about. It would be nursing without its soul. For a fuller appreciation of extant caring theories in nursing, the reader is referred to the rich and extensive literature already published elsewhere.

It is the very ordinariness of caring, both as a physical act and as a way of being, that contributes to the difficulties encountered in attempting to describe and define it. Caring is at once ubiquitous and specific – something commonplace, and yet a fine art that needs to be nurtured, developed, supported and valued. Much the same can be said for nursing – that its very familiarity contributes to its being undervalued and misunderstood, and yet, in a professional sense, nursing is seen as one of the most demanding interpersonal endeavours that can be undertaken, which is best accomplished when least noticed. A curious paradox.

The question that arises, however, is why now, at the tail end of the twentieth century, health-care professionals working with vulnerable and compromised members of the public should be so interested in the nature of caring. What is happening in the world around us that leaders of the helping professions see a need at this time to define, examine, promote and evaluate the significance of caring in the course of their work?

A second question related to the first and contingent on the picture that emerges from answering that question is, how does the public, that is, how does society value caring practices as defined by professionals? In what way does society show that it needs, expects and indeed wants its helping professionals to be caring? There is always a danger when professionals attempt to hijack common concepts and prevailing ideas that they are either obfuscating a fairly easily understood notion or, due to internal motives specific to their discipline, they are using the common and prevailing phenomena to prop up their own inadequacies. In times of low morale, it is not unusual for psychological rescue to be sought in the familiar and non-threatening areas of common agreement, cultural acceptance and historical certainty. Is caring a phenomenon so familiar that it can become a crutch and detractor of more serious woes? Or is caring the very heart and core of interpersonal professional work and the very essence of nursing – as some of its most outspoken advocates maintain (Leininger, 1984)? Is caring the hidden powerhouse and motivator of all work with and for the sick, vulnerable, broken and those in need of support? Or is caring merely another academic fad that will go the way of other notions long discarded by academicians, such as professionalism, advocacy or independence?

These questions need to be answered because, whereas with some other notions the long-term effect of academics toying with a concept and then throwing it aside is of little consequence, this might not always be the case. Thus nursing is a profession, whether or not nurse leaders or even the public agree on it. Advocacy as a social phenomenon has existed and will continue to exist whether or not nurses consciously endeavour to advocate for patients. Likewise, the independence of nursing will always remain a divisive issue, but nurses will continue to nurse and perceive their work as different from and/or complementary to that of medicine, physiotherapy and social work.

Therefore, in order to shed some light on the concept of caring as it is understood by nurse theorists, who by no means agree with each other, an overview of the main aspects of caring will be discussed. A few conceptual frameworks of the phenomenon will be presented, and finally examples of a few attempts to categorize and systematize these approaches will be given.

One of the most prevalent ways in which caring has been characterized is as a moral obligation. Whether as a member of the public or as a professional concerned with the promotion, restoration and maintenance of health, all individuals have a duty to care. The overriding human moral imperative to care is strong and deep seated, and is reflected in a myriad of forms in our society, from the highway code to the teaching of resuscitation skills to school-age children. For nurses, therefore, the moral imperative to care is both personal and professional.

Nurses are constrained to care by virtue of their code of practice. The professional caring of nurses is regulated by a registration requirement that advocates universal caring for all patients, pregnant women, vulnerable adults and members of the public who are in need of support, assistance or advice. All who come to nurses in need of their expert skills also have a right to expect a caring approach. Nurses care for all patients in a uniform manner unless, to paraphrase John Rawls' 'dictum of justice', more overall caring would be promoted by being selective about the extent and depth of caring shown to individual patients and clients (Rawls, 1971). This understanding of caring is enshrined in the code of conduct of the United Kingdom Central Council for Nurses and Midwives (UKCC). Although this requirement for nurses to be 'caring' is neither specific nor elaborated upon, it is regarded as an obligation to the extent that, where caring is seen to be wanting, nurses have been asked to account for their actions. Interestingly, the conflict of interests that can arise from caring for self, caring for members of the profession and caring for the public is not adequately addressed by the UKCC, although many complaints regarding nurses' actions stem directly from these conflicting moral demands and requirements. Several recent contentious statements by the UKCC, concerning the fate of nurses who did not adhere to the moral imperative to care for the public, owe much of their controversy to the fact that the UKCC Council for Professional Misconduct has a different set of values and caring priorities to the rest of the profession, not to mention the public. While professional caring for patients is seen as a non-negotiable deontological imperative, it is not a professional value of *supreme* importance in nursing; it is merely one of several moral values. Neither does the importance of caring for patients have a qualitatively different position in the hierarchy of moral values to the caring required of nurses towards each other (Keen, 1991). Caring is a professional moral imperative, but not *the* moral imperative.

Caring as an ethical way of being is a rather more broadly understood moral requirement. Here caring is both the result of moral development and the manifestation of professional and personal virtue. People are caring because their understanding of the requirements of social behaviour demands it, and because their personal conviction is that caring is a good virtue to cultivate. It is in fact the reflection of self-understanding and a promotion of the best interests of another. All the main philosophical movements of the West have advocated the promotion of caring, directly or indirectly, and it is certainly a major concern of moral philosophy. Modern philosophers have looked extensively at caring – what we care about, when we should care and even, in professional contexts, how we should care (Gaylin, 1976; Midgley, 1978; Noddings, 1984; Frankfurt, 1988; Warnock, 1992). Of all the various philosophies that address the issues of caring, existentialism and humanism are seen as the most relevant to nursing practice, even though the humanism referred to is usually poorly understood and articulated. Unfortunately, the existentialists cited are not necessarily the most appropriate exponents of caring philosophies, as these might be applied to nursing. However, for a more detailed and balanced analysis of this problem it would be necessary to read some existentialist philosophy (Warnock, 1970; Brykczyńska, 1995).

Apart from existentialist humanists, the early writings of Martin Heidegger are often cited. Heidegger, the German philosopher, who was an assistant to Edmund Husserl, the founder of modern phenomenology, wrote a classic work entitled *Being and Time*, which was first published in 1927. This early phenomenological work is the piece of philosophy most often cited by nurses.

In this early ontological work (which is concerned with the nature of 'being', specifically 'human' being), many nurse theorists who advocate a morality of caring find philosophical underpinnings for their ideas (Heidegger, 1962). The moral imperative to care, that owes much of its justification to a fundamentally deontological approach, is thus additionally buoyed up by an essentially ontological argument, which in turn owes most of its rationale to an interpretation of the ontological philosophy of Heidegger (Scudder, 1990). Advocates of Heideggerian ontological approaches to caring such as Jean Watson, Sister Simone Roach and Janice Morse, among many others, all interpret Heidegger's ontology in nursing terms. They see nursing as locating its being, that is, its essence, in the practice of caring. Caring, they claim, gives nursing its heart and soul. Without caring, nursing is but a collection of highly skilled tasks and endeavours – a recognizable body but without an animated soul. As Jean Watson (1988) notes, 'Caring is the moral ideal of nursing whereby the end is protection, enhancement, and preservation of human dignity' (see Chapter 3).

Sister Simone Roach (1992), elaborating upon her earlier treatise on caring, reaffirms her conviction that caring is the human mode of being and therefore also a uniquely appropriate means of professional caring. Roach maintains that, since all humans are capable of caring (as integrated and developed socio-moral beings), it is not surprising that nurses should identify with this aspect of their humanness and feel an additional need to analyse the nature of their professional caring. She states that

> Caring, as the human mode of being, entails the capacity or power to care, a capacity linked with and inseparable from our nature as human beings . . . . Caring is the actualization of the capacity or power to care.' (Roach, 1992, p. 47)

Madelaine Leininger, a pioneering nurse anthropologist, has developed a transcultural theory of caring in nursing, where she identifies commonalities and dissimilarities in human caring and suggests that far greater attention needs to be paid to the cultural dimension of caring motivations, acts and assumptions (Leininger, 1978). As a nurse-theorist, she is best known for her early nursing works on the nature of caring, in which she repeatedly and emphatically points out that, 'Caring is the essence of nursing' (Leininger, 1984). As part of her endeavour to identify caring acts in various cultures, she called upon nurses to start analysing caring actions and aspects of behaviour. However, this first wave of global definitions of the nature of caring was presented in a rather disorganized and chaotic manner.

More recently, nurses have attempted to analyse underlying caring constructs and various sub-themes emerging from the caring literature. This development is not surprising, and we now find ourselves in the second wave of professional literature, which is examining more closely specific aspects of caring, such as hope, empathy or comfort, and is less concerned with global definitions – which to some extent had launched the caring field of study. There is now a need to re-examine early caring theories in the light of recent specific caring epistemology and evaluative research studies.

It is therefore now possible not only to read and study how nurses perceive caring as a unique, identifiable professional and non-professional phenomenon but, in addition, to examine how caring occurs, what constituent aspects of human conduct are necessary for caring to be manifest, and the analysis of caring as experienced by both patients and nurses. The research is rich and varied, some of it representing particular identifiable perspectives, e.g. the work of Delores Gaut, who sees caring as a functional, intentional endeavour, and therefore in practice something that can be taught and transmitted (Gaut, 1984). Some research is examining the so-called 'lived experience' of caring for someone, or alternatively of being cared for, using a predominantly qualitative phenomenological research approach. This research methodology has been interpreted by the American social scientist, Dreyfus, and taken up and presented to nurses by nurse researchers such as Pat Benner and Janice Morse, from the qualitative school of nursing research. It is also now possible to study and analyse various individual constructs of caring, such as comfort, touch, support, hope, reciprocity, aspects of healing and, in a wider sense, works on spirituality, virtue, ethics of caring and moral development, and how these aspects of personhood impinge on caring. However, not all of the research is conducted with sufficient academic rigour to be of much permanent usefulness; there is evidence of some fashionable flag-waving, and already several outsiders looking at the work of nurses have voiced some reservations about the level of scholarship (Kruhse, 1995). However, concerns about the direction and nature of nursing research in this area are not unique to outsiders, and need to be confronted head on by nurses (Morse *et al.*, 1991; Radsma, 1994).

Janice Morse (1992), a nurse theorist and anthropologist, has looked at caring through the methodological perspective of phenomenology. As a senior advocate of this form of nursing research, she has herself contributed to the nursing debate on the nature of caring and has helped to shape contemporary professional thinking on the subject. In a joint paper written with a group of phenomenological nurse researchers she poses the question of whether it is time to start grouping the various extant nursing theories according to some coherent overview, in order to form a conceptual model of the various theories (Morse *et al.*, 1991). The authors have produced a picture of nurse-caring theories which categorizes the theories into five major approaches which, the authors note, are not as discrete in practice as the intellectual exercise would suggest. Thus they point out that caring can be conceptualized as a human trait, a moral imperative, an affect, an interpersonal interaction and an intervention.

Alison Kitson (1993), in the UK, has also looked at the problem of caring epistemology in an edited collection of essays which originated primarily from the works and concerns of the Nursing Institute in Oxford. She and her colleagues have attempted to address some of these issues. As Kitson noted in her introduction to formalizing concepts related to nursing and caring, 'In our individual search for understanding or making sense of the world around us, we rely consciously or unconsciously on our own conceptual maps to help us. . . . These concepts, whether we like it or not, or whether we know it or not, influence our everyday practice in numerous subtle and quite explicit ways . . .' (Kitson, 1993, p. 29). She therefore proceeds to demonstrate the need for a fresh examination and formation of a new picture of how traditional nursing theories based on prevailing philosophies and ideologies have shaped current thinking in nursing and are beginning to give direction to new research and caring theories. Rather than have separate, traditionally referred to 'models' of nursing, independent of contemporary 'caring' theories, there is a need to integrate the two approaches – if either have anything to offer and explain with regard to the practice of nursing. Certainly we can assume that it was not the intention of nurse theorists working from the needs-based, interactionist or holistic perspectives to denigrate the centrality of caring in nursing. It is possible, perhaps, that they took caring for granted, and assumed that it had to be present in nursing practice in the first place for, as Kitson noted, concepts influence everyday practice in subtle and not so subtle ways. The fact remains, however, that they did not overtly address the issue of caring. At the other end of the spectrum are the works of nurse theorists who are writing almost exclusively about caring, and yet who can be so global in their definitions that they could be referring to almost any of the helping professions, or indeed any profession. They are looking rather at the very nature and essence of caring – a philosophical exercise necessary for a social foundation of interpersonal works but not specific to nursing. The same observations concerning caring may hold true for the philosophical underpinnings of so-called lay-caring (Noddings, 1984).

Kitson has epitomized the caring imperative as a duty-based form of caring, exemplified by the exhortations of Florence Nightingale and still respected today, whenever we appreciate ethical acts which go above and beyond the ordinary, expected nursing norm. Here Kantian ethics are guided by virtue. Courage is still a powerful virtue, not overtly part of our nursing duty, but sometimes difficult to avoid in executing the nursing work that needs to be accomplished (Lanara, 1981; Fowler, 1986).

Kitson regards the caring theorists Leininger, Watson and Roach, who are concerned with the ontological nature of caring and consider caring as a therapeutic relationship, as being within the phenomenological approach to caring and influenced by twentieth century existentialists, in particular Heidegger and the American psychologist and philosopher, Milton Mayeroff (1971) (Leininger, 1978, 1984).

Interestingly, Kitson identifies a third group, represented by the nurse phenomenologist Patricia Benner (Benner and Wrubel, 1989). Members of this third group of theorists view caring as an ethical position, influenced by a virtue-ethics approach that overlaps, however, with the other two groups. In addition, the philosophy includes such humanistic approaches as those expressed by contemporary moral developmentalists such as Lawrence Kohlberg, his conceptual antagonist Carol Gilligan and the feminist philosopher N. Noddings. All of these academicians have heavily influenced recent approaches to nursing caring theories. However, it is Noddings' ideas concerning a feminist perspective on an ethic of care that have so profoundly affected the feminist approach to caring in nursing, an approach which is gaining momentum (Gilligan, 1982; Noddings, 1984; Kohlberg, 1986).

As Morse *et al.* (1991) have found, it is difficult to maintain these as discrete classifications, and although some nurses are content to justify their caring at a simple level, of duty to care, all other aspects and ways of looking at and living through caring will necessarily contain that core, which is specifically about the duty to care. Perhaps what we have here is not so much a series of matrixes or categorizations, as concentric circles, where all notions of caring stem from a common centre which, given the nature of our obligations towards patients, must in some way speak to a deontological imperative – that we ought to care. Emotive, affective and technical aspects of that imperative, to name but a few, all follow from that initial moral requirement. It is not a particularly picturesque approach, speaking as it does to the most fundamental level of our moral development, but that is precisely the point. We start our *professional* caring acts from the position that we have a duty to do so. However, there is nothing to stop us and much interpersonal growth to be gained from additionally developing a virtue ethic that supports that basic caring duty. Developing a conscience-based approach which identifies caring as *our* essential human mode of being does not exclude a duty-based professional approach. Certainly, these areas need much more reflection, research and academic attention than they have hitherto been accorded. There is much work that still needs to be done.

It is the intention of the authors of this book to present to the reader a collection of essays on the overall themes and constructs of caring as experienced in nursing practice. The authors look at caring from several perspectives and provide different insights on various issues within the caring concept – an eclectic approach to an elusive concept.

La Feu, speaking to the ailing King of France in Shakespeare's *All's Well that Ends Well* (Act II: Scene 1), notes that he has 'seen a medicine that's able to breath life into a stone.' I would like to think that that medicine is purposeful, competent and reflective caring, a potent elixir without which true healing cannot even start, and without which there is no purpose to life. Understanding and reflecting on the nature of caring can only help us to deliver this life-giving medicine.

References

Benner P and Wrubel J (1989) *The Primacy of Caring.* Addison-Wesley, Menlo Park, CA.

Brykczyńska G (1995) Humanism – a weak link in nursing theory? In Schober J and Hinchliff S (eds) *Towards Advanced Nursing Practice: Key Concepts for Healthcare*, pp. 111–32. Edward Arnold, London.

Fowler M (1986) Ethics without virtue. *Heart and Lung* 15, 528–30.

Frankfurt HG (1988) *The Importance of What We Care About: Philosophical essays.* Cambridge University Press, Cambridge.

Gaut D (1984) Development of a theoretically adequate description of caring. *Western Journal of Nursing Research* 5, 313–24.

Gaylin W (1976) *Caring.* Alfred A Knopf Publishers, New York, NY.

Gilligan C (1982) *In a Different Voice.* Harvard University Press, Cambridge, MA.

Heidegger M (1962) *Being and Time* (translated by Macquarrie J and Robinson E). SCM Press, London.

Keen P (1991) Caring for ourselves. In Neill RM and Watts R (eds) *Caring and Nursing: Explorations in Feminist Perspectives*, pp. 173–88. National League for Nursing, New York, NY.

Kitson A (ed.) (1993) *Nursing: Art and Science.* Chapman and Hall, London.

Kohlberg L (1986) Moral stages and moralization: the cognitive-developmental approach. In Lickona T (ed.) *Moral Development and Behaviour Theory: Research and Social Issues*, pp. 31–5. Holt, Rinehart and Winston, New York, NY.

Kruhse H (1995) Clinical ethics and nursing: 'yes' to caring, but 'no' to a female ethics of care. *Bioethics* 9, 207–19.

Lanara V (1981) *Heroism as a Nursing Value.* Sisterhood Evniki, Athens.

Leininger M (1978) *Transcultural Nursing: Concepts, Theories, and Practices.* John Wiley and Sons, Toronto.

Leininger M (1984) Caring: a central focus of nursing and healthcare services. In Leininger M (ed.) *Care: The Essence of Nursing and Health*, pp. 45–9. M Slack, Inc., Thorofare, NJ.

Mayeroff M (1971) *On Caring.* Harper and Row, Perennial Library, New York, NY.

Midgley M (1978) *Beast and Man: The Roots of Human Nature.* Methuen, London.

Morse J (ed.) (1992) *Qualitative Health Research.* Sage Publications Inc., Newbury Park, CA.

Morse JM, Bottorff J, Neander W and Solberg S (1991) Comparative analysis of conceptualizations and theories of caring. *Image: Journal of Nursing Scholarship* 23, 119–26.

Noddings N (1984) *Caring: a Feminine Approach to Ethics and Moral Education.* University of California Press, Berkeley, CA.

Radsma J (1994) Caring and nursing: a dilemma. *Journal of Advanced Nursing* 20, 444–9.

Rawls J (1971) *A Theory of Justice.* Harvard University Press, Cambridge, MA.

Roach Sister S (1992) *The Human Act of Caring: A Blue Print for the Health Professions,* *revised edn.* Canadian Hospital Association Press, Ottawa, Ontario.

Scudder JR (1990) Dependent and authentic care: implications of Heidegger for nursing care. In Leininger M and Watson J (eds) *The Caring Imperative in Education,* pp. 59–66. National League for Nursing, New York, NY.

Warnock M (1970) *Existentialism.* Oxford University Press, Oxford.

Warnock M (1992) *The Uses of Philosophy.* Blackwell, Oxford.

Watson J (1988) *Nursing: Human Science and Human Care. A Theory of Nursing.* National League for Nursing, New York, NY.

Further reading

Brykczyńska G (1992) Caring – a dying art? In Jolley M and Brykczyńska G (eds) *Nursing – the Challenge to Change,* pp. 1–45. Edward Arnold, London.

Brykczyńska G (1995) Reflective practice: an analysis of nursing wisdom. In Jolley M and Brykczyńska G (eds) *Nursing: Beyond Tradition and Conflict,* pp. 9–28. Mosby, London.

Taylor B (1994) *Being Human: Ordinariness in Nursing.* Churchill Livingstone, Edinburgh.

Van Hooft S (1995) *Caring: an Essay in the Philosophy of Ethics.* University Press of Colorado, Niwot, CO.

2

The historical tradition of care

Ann Bradshaw

Societies have always striven to look after the weak, infirm and chronically disabled, and when they fail to do so, they present a less than human aspect of their approach to social awareness. This chapter examines the long tradition of Western culture in caring for its more vulnerable members, and reminds the reader of the strong Judaeo-Christian religious legacy that has been inherited by the modern nursing profession. Just as an awareness of family roots is important for a feeling of personal belonging, so an awareness of the historical roots of nursing is important for a feeling of maturity for modern nurses. The roots of nursing have grounded the profession in a firm tradition of enlightened and deliberate caring – an informed compassion. However, this tradition of caring is not just another reflection of the cultural and religious norms of previous centuries that is irrelevant to modern nursing. Caring was considered to be central to nursing practice as it was based on an understanding of moral development deemed to be necessary for good nursing practice. Likewise, today, in order to promote a wise caring praxis we too should pay more attention to the ethical development of nurses.

Introduction

In 1967 a book entitled *Sans Everything* was published. This was a direct result of a letter in *The Times* 2 years earlier, which protested against the cruelty and neglect of elderly patients in certain hospitals. The author, Barbara Robb, suggests that nurses were recruited who came to see their defenceless patients as the sources of their disagreeable and hard work. The nurses vented their frustration on these vulnerable patients, who were unable to complain for fear that this would make matters worse, and even relatives suppressed complaints out of concern for the patients. *Sans Everything* provides detailed statements from nurses themselves of the cruelty, callousness, filth and depersonalization that they were witnessing.

Patients were deprived of their dignity and humanity, roughly, even brutally, handled, and left to sit all day in tea-stained and urine-soaked clothes. Let me quote just one of the numerous examples:

> Bath mornings took place twice a week. Forty-four patients had to be bathed, and this was a nightmare. The sister in charge showed me how it was to be done. I had always at least eight patients stripped naked. One was put into each bath, while the others jostled one another. The incontinent patients often wetted the piles of clean towels and clothes on the urine-saturated floors . . . I was astonished and horrified by the way in which trained staff discussed the patients in front of them, as if they were stone deaf as well as confused. I saw one woman called up to the sister's table in the day room and made to pull up her clothes to show that she had wet knickers. This in front of a male cleaner who, poor lad, was most embarrassed. The patient put out her hand and touched the sister's white apron and said, 'You may be white on top, sister, but not underneath'.
>
> (Robb, 1967, p. 38)

How could this happen? What causes one person to treat another with such a lack of humanity? Eminent professionals suggested factors such as low professional status, inadequate knowledge, poor staffing levels and weak leadership, and undoubtedly these contributed to low morale and the lack of care. But are these factors a sufficient explanation? In the words of the patient, what makes the nurse 'white underneath'? And if we turn the question round the other way, what makes us *care*? In the Afterword to *Sans Everything*, M David Enoch, a consultant psychiatrist, suggests that the issue is a moral and religious problem:

> [The elderly] may be a weak and unattractive group; economically unproductive; scientifically and psychologically uninteresting – 'Ready for the Scrapheap'. But they cannot be ignored. Nor is it sufficient to talk about them. Our civilization will be judged not only on our social and material progress but also on the provision made for the weakest in our midst . . . Our concern and relationship with our fellow-men must surely be a moral and religious problem. ('For as much as ye have done it unto the least of these, ye have done it unto me').
>
> (Enoch, 1967, p. 139)

This lack of care for the weak and sick in society was precisely the problem that Nightingale sought to address in the mid-nineteenth century. 'We see the nurses drinking, we see the neglect at night owing to their falling asleep. Where women undertake so toilsome an office, for hire, and not for love, it cannot be otherwise' (Nightingale, 1851, p. 15). Indeed, Dickens himself, who immortalized the pre-Nightingale paid nurse in his characters Sarah Gamp and Betsey Prig, commented in 1867, in a preface to *Martin Chuzzlewit*, 'I think it not the least among the instances of their mismanagement, that Mrs Betsey Prig was a fair specimen of a Hospital Nurse; and that the Hospitals, with their means and friends, should have left it to private humanity and enterprise to enter on an attempt to improve that class of persons – since, greatly improved through the agency of *good* women' (Dickens in Kosky, 1989, p. 210) (my italics). The work of care, as Nightingale believed and we shall further explore, could not occur with women of 'bad character', for it depended on more than contractual ties; care was the result of the principle which she calls 'love', and rested in the 'goodness' of the carer.

However, the following question arises. Are the sad cases detailed in *Sans Everything*, as well as the stories of paid, contracted and uncaring nurses brought to life by Dickens, just anachronisms from past ages? We are warned against holding any such notions. For even in spring 1994 the United Kingdom Central Council for Nursing, Midwifery and Health Visiting (1994a) has detailed cases of gross physical and verbal abuse of elderly patients in nursing homes by registered nurses. We need to remember, too, that such cases of cruelty are extreme. A nurse does not need to be cruel to be without heart. If nurses are capable of such abuse, then they, even *we*, may be capable of coldness of heart and a poverty of compassion. We do not need to reach the extreme of cruelty to provide our patients with care that lacks warmth or kindness. This issue of humane care is as relevant for us today as it was in the past. And perhaps we might learn lessons from our past in order to help us move forward in the future. For we are reminded that the nature of care, involving our attitudes and responses to other human beings, depends on the moral foundation of goodness.

The moral dimension of care

I suggest that our current concern with 'quality' in health care is dependent on the values that underpin our attitudes, individually and corporately, when we care for patients and clients. This is dawningly realized by the Chief Medical Officer, Kenneth Calman (1993, p. 1), when he writes that quality is related to values: 'It is then necessary to define more clearly what these values are, and to set them out in a way that shows how to improve quality. Values are the key to many things in health and health care.' For Calman, as he himself states, his eyes were opened through reading Robert Pirsig's *Zen and the Art of Motorcycle Maintenance* and *Lila: an Enquiry into Morals*. However, surely it is self-evident that quality in health care depends on underlying values. The attitude of the carer, the way he or she expresses care and responds to the person who needs care, that unquantifiable quality of genuine compassion, kindness, gentleness and understanding alongside skill, knowledge and competence, are the very essence of good health care. Surely this is a truism that we all know. Yet it is precisely here that nurses are trying to reach consensus, as nursing writers seek to articulate and delineate this elusive quality of care.

And perhaps we should not be surprised at the problem nursing has in reaching a consensus in defining 'care', for the term 'care' itself seems to have grown nebulous. So, for example, we read in the 'Statement of Purpose of the Council' (UKCC, 1994b) that the 'Values of the Council' are 'Care' 'Protect' and 'Honour' (*sic*). And we need to ask the UKCC the following moral question. Does not the concept of care subsume within it the values of protection and honour? To care is to protect and to honour. Or rather, can care be care without offering protection or honouring trust? Are not these values or virtues inseparable? We must assume that the UKCC thinks that they can be separated. We can no longer assume that nursing holds a universal understanding of care, and so it has become a major nursing concern to define a moral foundation and thus a universal meaning for nursing today.

Peter Jarvis, Professor of Continuing Education at Surrey University, in his response to a nursing paper on patient-centred health care, has concluded that the nurse is 'the guardian of a tradition about the meaning of nursing into which new nurses are inducted'. Ending with the words of Martin Buber that 'Education worthy of the name is essentially education of character', Jarvis suggests that 'the character of the nurse is as important as the knowledge that she possesses' (Jarvis, 1996). Jarvis's ending may serve as our starting point. For although Jarvis may not have been aware of it, this word 'character' was used by Nightingale as the primary moral force underpinning the good nurse. This was what made her, in the phrase used earlier, 'white underneath'. We shall therefore focus our discussion on this motivating force behind the personality of the carer, the nature of the nurse's 'character' and its relationship to the moral dimension of care. In order to do this, we shall look at contemporary ideas about the caring character and compare these with the traditional view of what makes nurses caring.

The character of the carer

Before we make this excursion into the traditional moral basis for nursing care, we need briefly to consider current positions on the philosophical basis of care. The view expressed by Noddings (1984), which is similar to the ethical approach adopted by Benner (1991), serves as a relevant example of a modern view, that caring is a particularly feminine trait derived from feminine emotional qualities. The carer becomes fulfilled when she becomes involved in caring relationships through engrossment and motivational displacement. This is a situationist position. There are no universal moral norms or principles of care. Each relationship is unique. In order to support her position, Noddings is drawn to the theology of Buber (1958). She finds, in his concept of the I-Thou relationship, the basis for a warm and relational human understanding of caring.

Noddings rejects both the rationalism of utilitarian ethics, that care is for a particular purpose, and the Kantian ethic of duty. She finds the Kantian rational approach to the concept of care cold and unfeeling, and Iris Murdoch would agree with her. Murdoch's criticism of Kant in *Metaphysics as a Guide to Morals* (1993) highlights the weaknesses of a cold and rational morality:

> Moreover acting rightly toward another person does not necessarily, in fact more often does not, involve face-to-face encounters. There is here a contrast of styles which can be comprehensively illustrated in everyday terms. One man does good by stealth, attends carefully to the situation of others, sees their needs, helps them without close involvement, even anonymously, admonishes indirectly, by implication and example, and shuns close encounter. Only in rare situations would it be a duty, or indeed possible, to achieve complete mutual understanding. Another man prefers to draw people close to him, to have confessions, frank meetings, warmth and friendship, to give support by voice and presence. No doubt the afflicted human race needs both of these philanthropists. There is an essential area of coldness in morality, as there is an essential area of warmth. Seen in Kantian context, the I-Thou concept can seem (by contrast) thrilling and dramatic, readily compromised by various self-regarding consolations. It holds out a promise of experience and ever-available company.
>
> (Murdoch, 1993, p. 470)

However, Noddings' position has three weaknesses. First, it fails to acknowledge the common humanity in caring, that care is not predominantly gender-specific. Men also care, and know about care, as Buber himself shows. Indeed, as feminists such as Dalley (1988) and Salvage (1985) argue, this view, that women are by nature the carers in society, in their opinion perpetuates inequality. Women are disempowered and relegated to subservient domesticity, while men are empowered as rational providers. The second weakness of Noddings' argument is highlighted by the 'carers' in *Sans Everything*. Here were women who did not care. Noddings' approach to caring focuses on caring relationships between family and friends, but does not consider relationships between people without bonds of natural affinity, such as nurses and patients. Here we see highlighted the very arbitrariness of using personal feelings as a basis for caring. What happens to 'care' when the 'carer' does not feel like caring? The third weakness of Noddings' position is described by Blustein (1991). Her notion of caring does not distinguish the good or bad of what is cared about – the moral content of care.

This is the crucial point for a profession such as nursing, which necessarily rests on an unequal relationship between nurse and patient by virtue of the patient's need and vulnerability. For Buber, the moral base and norm of care rests in the theological understanding of *agape*. This is the foundation and objectivity of the I-Thou relationship. However, Noddings rejects this theological base. She cuts away the root of her position, leaving it hanging in the air. But as Buber (1990) argued against Carl Rogers, this root is necessary for maintaining the objectivity of care against mere emotion, and so sustaining a genuineness and mutuality in a professional relationship where the person being cared for is in a more vulnerable position than the carer. The moral nature of care depends on this root. Indeed, this was precisely Warnock's (1988) criticism of Kant, that his moral imperative presupposed the theological assumptions of the Judaeo-Christian tradition in which he was brought up; and it was against this that Nietzsche (1954) wrote. If we cut away the theological foundation of morality, then morality is nothing more than our own personal preferences and our own will to power. And if this is so, why should we care? And about what? Hence the moral basis and content of care is a question that nursing needs to address.

The question then for us as nurses is where our duty of care comes from. How do we know what it is to care, and is the meaning of care the same for us all? (We have already seen earlier, with reference to the UKCC, that we cannot assume that it is.) This brings us not just to a question of how we should care, but why we should care at all. Why should we care not only for the cheerful, helpful and grateful patient or client, but also for people who may be unattractive, ungrateful, unhygienic, awkward and demanding? What is the moral impetus to care? This is our first question. And the second question is related to it: how should we care? In order to help us find an answer to these questions I believe we need to look at history, to our tried and tested tradition, and find out what the moral basis and thus the content and direction of care has been in our nursing heritage. How and in what ways did the profession of nursing arise, and what inspired women and sometimes men to care for people who were often the derelicts of society? The answer will be found in the sentence quoted earlier by Enoch: 'For as much as ye have done it unto the least of these, ye have done it unto me.'

The traditional moral basis of care

As the sociologist Robert Dingwall (1977, p. 31) has written, the traditional model of nursing in Britain until the 1960s has been what he calls a 'Nightingale model', the basis of which was vocation. Derived from a laicization of the religious calling and the religious order, it was an approach to care that demanded a total commitment. 'Religious inspiration was an important motivating force in the lives of many nurses.' Referring to the work of Katherine Williams, Dingwall suggests that the ideology of 'Vocation' (*sic*) dignified the idea of service, self-abasement and the performance of the 'menial tasks' of care. We shall need to look later at such current interpretations of this vocational attitude. For Dingwall himself takes a critical and even pejorative interpretation of this vocational approach which is in line with much contemporary nursing revisionism. We cannot ignore this criticism, both because of its justification and because of its effect on current nursing ideology, and we shall consider these views later in the chapter. For the present, suffice it to say that Dingwall has offered us a glimpse of the moral basis that underpinned the traditional nursing model of care.

Nightingale, the great exemplar of nursing, provides a useful starting place for us, for in her we might see gathered together both the tradition of care that preceded her as well as that to which she gave new life. In fact, we may be able to claim, with some justification, that Nightingale personified the traditional nursing ethic of care. Nightingale's vision of nursing grew out of a profound faith in God which rooted and grounded her life. Called by God on four separate occasions, Nightingale responded personally in her own life by eschewing the comfortable life of a wealthy gentlewoman to which she had been brought up. She sailed to the Crimea, worked among dying, wounded and filthy soldiers, lived in appalling squalor and freezing temperatures, because she was living out the biblical commandment of love. She saw the brutalized soldier as a child of God, and treated him not as a savage animal, but as a person beloved by his creator, and in this she encompassed the whole moral basis for care. From these beginnings grew her own understanding of God's relationship to human beings and the implication of this for nursing. She spent her life exploring this theology in complex and often muddled writing, but also by putting it into practical action through the nurses that trained in her name and with her principles.

As Quinn and Prest (1987, p. xxii), Fellows of Balliol College, Oxford, discovered when they examined the enormous correspondence between Nightingale and Benjamin Jowett, the eminent nineteenth-century theologian and Master of Balliol, 'Florence Nightingale's life was predicated upon her faith in God ...' She believed in a religious approach to social problems, and in this she mirrored very similar ideas that underpinned the political movement of Christian socialism. Nurses trained at the Nightingale school at St Thomas's did not undertake private work, but were sent out as 'missionaries for cleanliness' to the great London teaching hospitals and workhouse infirmaries of the big cities. We are reminded that Nightingale's approach was revolutionary in the sacrifice it called for from its nurses, for hospitals in the nineteenth century were dangerous institutions, despised by the rich, and used only by the poor. 'The stronger the sense of vocation a Nightingale nurse possessed, the more likely she was to be brought into contact with patients who could tell her what life was like at the bottom of society, in overcrowded houses, among men engaged in casual labour and women worn out by child-rearing.' For one such Nightingale nurse, Agnes Jones, her profound evangelical Christian faith led her to work in a Liverpool workhouse, and eventually brought about her own death from cholera contracted in the workhouse (Jones, 1871).

For Nightingale, as she wrote many times in addresses to her probationer nurses at St Thomas's, the quality of the nurse's care depended at the most fundamental level on the moral character of the nurse. This recalls Buber's words quoted earlier by Jarvis: 'Education worthy of the name is essentially education of *character*' (my emphasis). If we seek to understand exactly what Nightingale meant by this word, we can do no better than look at her explanation in her own words, chosen as the final quotation from all her vast writings by Sir Edward Cook to sum up his two-volume seminal biography of her life:

> Live your life while you have it. Life is a splendid gift. There is nothing small in it. For the greatest things grow by God's law out of the smallest. But to live your life, you must discipline it. You must not fritter it away in 'fair purpose, erring act, inconstant will', but must make your thought, your words, your acts all work to the same end, and that end not self but God. This is what we call CHARACTER [*sic*].
>
> (Cook, 1913b, p. 434)

Thus, for Nightingale, the notion of character was very much of a moral nature and concerned the unity of the individual within a purpose of life. 'A woman cannot be a good and intelligent nurse without being a good and intelligent woman'. This formed the whole basis of what she understood to be the purpose of nurse training:

> To obey *is* to understand orders, and to understand orders really is to obey. A nurse does not know how to do what she is told without such 'training' as enables her to understand what she is told; or without such moral and disciplinary 'training' as enables her to give her whole self to obey. A woman cannot be a good and intelligent nurse without being a good and intelligent woman. Therefore, what 'training' signifies in the wide sense, what makes a *good training-school*, what moral and disciplinary 'training' means, and how it is to be attained, are to be clearly understood.
>
> (Nightingale, 1882, p. 1039)

If we consider her words, we can see that Nightingale was not advocating a blind obedience to authority as nursing revisionists now assume, in the sense, as Dingwall (1977, p. 31) puts it, of 'total submission to authority', but rather an obedience born out of understanding the moral obligation demanded of the whole self in service. This is because she saw obedience as the sense of understanding that develops through moral and technical training or education. This becomes clearer if we examine Nightingale's detailed description of what such training entails. Practically, she believes that this involves observation and trained reflection:

> Observation tells *how* the patient is; reflection tells, *what* is to be done; training tells *how* it is to be done. Training and experience are, of course, necessary to teach us, too, *how* to observe, *what* to observe, *how* to think, *what* to think. Observation tells us the fact; reflection the meaning of the fact. Reflection needs training as much as observation.
>
> (Nightingale, 1882, p. 1039)

Nightingale proceeds to detail the content of the nurse's training. This included clinical lectures from hospital professors on chemistry, anatomy, physiology, medicine and surgery, to be tested by written and oral examinations, as well as practical and technical training under the head nurse or 'sister' with special emphasis on the moral qualities of the probationer that would be necessary in her ward work. Nightingale the statistician saw the supreme importance of the scientific, technical and practical knowledge needed by the nurse, objectively examined and tested, while Nightingale the woman of faith realized that, above all, the nurse's care rested in the moral quality of the practitioner.

This is made clear in many of her letters to her probationer nurses at St Thomas's, and was the reason for her dispute with Mrs Bedford Fenwick over the registration of nursing. As Nightingale wrote in a letter in 1888:

> Has not everyone who has experience of the world been struck by this? You may have the most admirable circumstances and organizations and examinations and certificates – yet if the individual allows herself to sink to a lower level, it is all but a 'tinkling cymbal' for her. It is how the circumstances are worked that signifies. Circumstances are opportunities. Rules may become a dead letter. It is the Spirit of them that 'giveth life'. It is the individual, inside, that counts – the level she is upon which tells. The rest is only the outward shell or envelope. She must become 'a rule of thought' to herself through the Ruler. . . . It is, again, what the individual nurse *is* and can do during her *living* training and *living* work that signifies – not what she is certified for, like a steam boiler which is certified to stand so much pressure of work. She may have gone through a first rate course – plenty of examinations. And we may find nothing inside. It may be the difference between a Nurse Nursing, and a Nurse reading a book on Nursing. Unless it bear fruit, it is all gilding and veneering; the reality is not there.

If we look again at the sentence, 'She may have gone through a first rate course – plenty of examinations. And we may find nothing inside,' we may be reminded of the patient quoted earlier who criticized the cruel and heartless sister for being 'white on top but not underneath'. We also see clearly the resonances with the discussion pursued by the moral philosopher Mary Midgley. She suggests that the core of the human being, his 'heart', is where the person's priorities are formed, and she continues:

> How then does this centre relate to the mind or brain? Here too we can choose between a wider and a narrower use. We certainly can contrast the mind or brain sharply with the heart, as I did just now in speaking of the medical student. *He may have a first-class mind – meaning that he always passes exams well – without any necessary consequences about his heart or character.*
>
> (Midgley, 1981, p. 2) (my emphasis)

However, while Midgley's use of 'character' seems very similar to that meant by Nightingale, we cannot assume that they have the same understanding of what constitutes 'character'. Nightingale is clear that the nurse's warmed heart rests in the biblical, New Testament values expressed in the Sermon on the Mount: 'A really good nurse must needs be of the highest class of character . . . a good nurse should be the "Sermon on the Mount" in herself' (Nightingale, 1882, p. 1048). So Nightingale talks about the nurse offering her patient a kind of love or *agape* that puts the patient's needs first:

Thinking of her patient and not of herself; 'tender over his occasions' or wants, cheerful and kindly, patient, ingenious and *feat* . . . A patient wants according to his wants, and not according to any nurse's theory of his wants or 'occasions' . . . The nurse must have simplicity and a single eye to the patient's good. She must make no demand upon the patient for reciprocation, for acknowledge- ment or even perception of her services; since the best service a nurse can give *is* that the patient shall scarcely be aware of any – shall perceive her presence only by perceiving that he has *no* wants. The nurse must always be kind, but never emotional. The patient must find a real, not forced or 'put on', centre of calmness in his nurse. To call upon a patient by emotion for emotion is the most cruel, because useless, demand upon his strength. It is asking him to bear your troubles and your anxiety as well as his own.

Here we see that this moral quality of character is not merely emotional, but that it is a self-sacrificing devotion derived from what Wesley called the 'warmed heart', and indeed this idea of care as love or charity is the prime moral commandment of the Judaeo-Christian tradition, profoundly differentiating it from previous moral traditions. Thus, for example, Aristotle's account of human nature expressed in the virtues has no place for humility or charity which, as we see clearly from her writing, Nightingale considered to be fundamental virtues for the good nurse. As MacIntyre writes:

For The New Testament not only praises virtues of which Aristotle knows nothing – faith, hope and love – and says nothing about virtues such as *phronêsis* which are crucial for Aristotle, but it praises at least one quality as a virtue which Aristotle seems to count as one of the vices relative to magnanimity, namely humility.

(MacIntyre, 1985, p. 182)

Perhaps from our viewpoint at the very end of the twentieth century it is easy to overlook the revolutionary significance of Nightingale's position as to what lies at the heart of a good nurse. For Nightingale, as Dingwall (1977) suggests, developed her nursing philosophy amid the regimentation of army discipline. It would therefore not have been surprising if she had emphasized the leadership characteristics of the army leader in formulating her theory of what constituted a good nursing leader, and so stressed skills such as leadership and man management, which she herself undoubtedly possessed. While these were no doubt important to her, what was of much more fundamental signi- ficance was the moral quality of the nurse. As we see, she stresses the character that is 'tender' and 'kind', and genuinely so, not 'put on' or derived from mere emotional feelings, and above all found in humility and self-effacement. Nightingale turned the values of her contemporaries upside down. Nurses were not to seek status, but rather to aim for service. Nursing was not to seek professionalization as an end in itself, but rather to maintain the ideals of the vocation. Nightingale saw the vital significance of such personal attributes because of her own intrinsic beliefs and values about the nature of the person.

Thus the kind of moral character Nightingale is advocating rests not in the rational will (with Kant), nor in the emotions (with the situationists such as

Noddings), but in the unity of the individual in relationship to his fellow man, because of its religious basis in creation. According to William Temple (1942), this was a basis for freedom, fellowship and service, and it is because of this basis in the created order that we see clearly that the character of care embraces an inextricable relationship to cure. Patient-centred care directed at the whole person requires the appropriation of the methods and understandings of science and technology. As Titmuss writes (1963, p. 129): 'With all her intense preoccupation with means, the design of hospital wards, the planning of hospital space, sanitation, the proper use of record forms and so forth, Florence Nightingale never lost sight of the fundamental needs of the patient.' This was because, for Nightingale, the patient-centred nature of care, the moral dimension of care, was not merely an emotion or motivation of the will, but rather the universal activity of love grounded in a rational, ordered creation, the laws of which hold within them the potential to prevent disease and cure illness. Indeed, as the historian Sir Keith Thomas (1973), the physician Lord Walton (1990) and the philosopher Professor Roger Trigg (1993) all point out, the Judaeo-Christian understanding of order in creation formed the foundation for the growth and development of natural science.

However, we might also pause to reflect here that, as important as Nightingale considered science to be, she firmly believed that it formed an inadequate basis for care. As she constantly repeated in her many writings, if the moral character of the nurse were lost, the future of nursing would be imperilled. This was why she was so fearful of professionalization. Even in her time, Nightingale foresaw Weber's (Gerth and Mills, 1991) thesis of the routinization of charisma – his argument that bureaucratization and institutionalization over time eventually suppressed the essential spirit through which the endeavour was founded. As her convictions state:

> But I do entirely and constantly believe that the *religious motive* is essential for the highest kind of nurse. There are such disappointments, such sickenings of the heart, that they can only be borne by the feeling that one is called to the work by God, that it is a part of His work, that one is a fellow-worker with God. 'I do not ask for success,' said dear Agnes Jones, even while she was taking every human means to ensure success, 'but that the will of God may be done in me and by me'.
>
> (Cook, 1913, p. 271)

So she believed in the influence of the individual founder; what Weber might have called the 'charismatic leader', Nightingale saw as the vocational, spiritual call of the individual to service.

Like Weber, she saw the institution developed from this original foundation gradually losing its spiritual heart:

> 'For my part,' she said, 'I think that people should always be Founders. And this is the main argument against Endowments. While the Founder is there, his or her work will be done, not afterwards. The Founder cannot foresee the evils

which will arise when he is no longer there. Therefore let him not try to establish an Order. This has been most astonishingly true with the Order of the Jesuits as founded by S. Ignatius Loyola, and with S. Vincent de Paul's Soeurs de la Charité. It is quite immeasurable the breadth and length which now separates the spirit of those Orders from the spirit of their Founders.'

(Cook, 1913, p. 271)

(This might later be seen to be contradicted by Nightingale's praise of the Sisters of Charity.)

We shall shortly look back to the tradition of care preceding Nightingale to see how justified Nightingale's words might be deemed, but (and we cannot go into this here) her words and their resonances with Weber's thesis strike chords with what James and Field (1992) have recently argued to be the bureaucratization and routinization that have developed in the modern hospice movement. Here, too, the spiritual values of Cicely Saunders, the founder of the modern hospice movement, who herself built on a long tradition of Christian care for the dying, may now be seen to be becoming ever more marginal. Moreover, according to Midgley (1981, p. 57) it is this kind of 'personal example' that '*can* alter standards' and 'in fact, it is probably the central method of doing so. It is not glamorous and seldom receives medals . . .'. However, it is precisely this abstract moral quality that is so susceptible to the forces of bureaucratization and the idea that the components of caring behaviour, caring skills, techniques and attitudes can somehow be measured and codified. Nightingale and Saunders embodied the morality of care. They lived it out themselves, not as a standard or technique, but as an outpouring of their hearts, and so set a personal example for those who followed in their work.

However, they too followed in a tradition of 'charismatic', inspired men and women, whose lives were an example to them, and both Nightingale (1851) and Saunders (1986) were very well aware of the significance, nature and influence of this spiritual tradition of care on their own work and lives. Nightingale makes this clear in her booklet about Kaiserswerth on the Rhine, the institution for the practical training of deaconesses, where she stayed, and which helped to form her conception of nursing. This institution, founded by Pastor Fliedner, a Lutheran Pietist Clergyman, included a reformatory prison, an infant school, an orphanage and a hospital. Fliedner, who had himself been influenced by the faith of Elizabeth Fry, whom he had visited in England, developed the Kaiserswerth Institution as a Christian model of care. And it is the effect of this moral basis on the quality of care for the sick, weak and infirm that so impresses Nightingale:

Let such as feel this [women who feel the need for moral or spiritual work] go to Kaiserswerth, and see the delicacy, the cheerfulness, the grace of Christian kindness, the moral atmosphere, in short, which may be diffused through a hospital, by making it one of God's schools, where both patients and nurses come to learn of Him.

We are aware of the difficulty and the disgust, which would attend a woman who wished to learn in a hospital, as commonly conducted. None such need deter her from visiting Kaiserswerth. First, the kindness of the sisters in imparting their own knowledge is as remarkable, when contrasted with the jealousy of nurses and surgeons, in general, as the refinement with which it is done. The Pastor's spirit seems to pervade the whole sisterhood.

(Nightingale, 1851, p. 19)

At Kaiserswerth, Nightingale saw a model of care that contrasted sharply with the contemporary model of English nursing, rational care without a heart, performed by paid servants, 'nurses' who were mere tools of cold philanthropy. The vocational motive that inspired the caring practice at Kaiserswerth, although Lutheran and therefore Protestant, was the same force that was already at work among the Roman Catholic Sisters of Charity, the nursing order founded by St Vincent de Paul in France, in the previous century.

More labourers are wanted, and more will come. If this may be their future, the fear of becoming 'old maids' will disappear; if they may be instructed how to become the active 'handmaids of the Lord,' what life can they desire more? That English women can work, and work successfully in this cause, is proved by the Roman Catholic Sisters of Charity. Shall the Roman Catholic Church do all the work? Has not the Protestant the same Lord, who accepted the services not only of men, but also of women? The harvest is ripe. Where are the sick and the poor wanting? Let those women of England, who sit in busy idleness, look at Germany. There are your sisters all at work, Christ in their midst. Let Him not say, I have called my English handmaidens, but they would not answer. I stood at their door and knocked, but they would not open.

(Nightingale, 1851, p. 32)

Historical origins for the moral tradition of care

Nightingale looks back to the moral and spiritual tradition of care that originated through biblical precept and was established in the early church.

For every want we can always find a divine supply. And accordingly, we see, in the very first times of Christianity, an apostolical institution for the employment of woman's powers directly in the service of God. We find them engaged as 'servants of the Church'. We read, in the Epistle to the Romans, of a 'Deaconess,' as in the Acts of the Apostles, of 'Deacons'. Not only men were employed in the service of the sick and poor, but also women. In the fourth century, St Chrysostom speaks of forty Deaconesses at Constantinople. We find them in the Western Church as late as the eighth, – in the Eastern, as the twelfth century. . . . 'Many chose,' it is said, 'the single state, not because they expected thereby to reach a super-eminent degree of holiness, but that they might be the better able to care for the sick and the young.'

(Nightingale, 1851, p. 8)

The historian Adolf von Harnack reiterates this same conception of care:

'I was sick and ye visited me . . . As ye have done it unto one of the least of these my brethren, ye have done it unto me.' In these words the founder of Christianity set the love that tends the sick in the centre of his religion, laying it on the hearts of all his disciples. Primitive Christianity carried it in her heart; she also carried it out in practice.

(Harnack, 1961, p. 120)

As Harnack writes, this conception of love growing out of the heart and motivating care for the sick and derelict of humanity was a radical departure from the general attitude to the weak in the Graeco-Roman world.

The Greek nursing Professor, Vassiliki Lanara, has explored the influence of Greek and Christian ideas on the development of nursing, particularly during the Byzantine period. She writes:

Christianity created a climate very favourable to the development of nursing. Love and service to one's fellow men were predominant values in the Byzantine culture. Nursing as loving care evolved from the Christian religion. The parable of the Good Samaritan and Christ's teaching: 'I was sick and ye visited me' (St Matthew 25 v. 36) constituted the basis for patient care in the Byzantine era.

(Lanara, 1976, p. 49)

What is not clear from Lanara's writing, however, is the question as to how radically the Christian conception of philanthropy departed from the Greek Hippocratic tradition. Lord Walton, in his 1990 Harveian Oration, has described the Greek concept of *philia* as love for man in the abstract, while *technie*, or the practice of medicine embodied in the Hippocratic tradition, referred to a love for the art of healing. He believes that it was the Christian conception of love as *agape* that transformed the Greek practice of medicine, and he cites the example of the Greek attitude to incurable illness, which was not addressed by Greek medicine, for it was believed that such illnesses which could not be healed were not pleasing to the gods, who required health above all else. Constantelos (1968) supports this interpretation, and explores this issue in depth. He writes that the Greek notion of *philanthropia* was broadened and deepened in both theory and practice under the impact of the Christian teaching of *agape*.

As the evidence indicates, one can clearly discern that in the early Christian societies of both the East and the West philanthropia had assumed an integrated and far-reaching meaning. The term was used to describe man's love for the totality of humanity. Its application was directed to even the humblest among men. Philanthropia appropriated the meaning of selfless love and willing sacrifice. It was extended to the underprivileged, as it proclaimed freedom, equality and brotherhood, transcending sex, race, and national boundaries. Thus, conclusively, philanthropia was not limited to equals, allies and relatives, nor to citizens and civilized men, as was most often the case in ancient Greece. Christianity adopted the Greek concept of philanthropia but it went further in its application.

(Constantelos, 1968, p. 16)

This same inspiration is recorded by Clay (1966) in her work *The Mediaeval Hospitals of England*. She writes:

> While we are justly proud of our institutions for the amelioration of the lot of the infirm and destitute, we are apt to forget that they are not the outcome of any modern philanthropic movement, but are rather England's inheritance for above a thousand years.
>
> (Clay, 1966, p. xvii)

She records a picture of mediaeval England which, despite a general population that was smaller than that of London when Clay was writing, contained more than 750 charitable institutions apart from monasteries and friaries committed to relief of the body and refreshment of the soul.

> The fact proves that clergy and laity were battling bravely with social problems. There existed a sense of responsibility, causing real charitable effort, although mediaeval methods may appear mistaken in the light of modern scientific and economic principles.
>
> (Clay, 1966, p. xviii)

While Clay points out that in the mediaeval religious mind, faith and love predominated over skill and science, we need to remind ourselves that it was the same religious frame of mind that, as Thomas (1973) has shown, laid the groundwork for natural science and thus provided the soil for the Renaissance, the Reformation and pioneering medical discoveries and, indeed, opened the way for Descartes' rationalism and the Enlightenment itself. So, as we have seen with Nightingale, the religious frame of mind was uniquely able to hold faith and love together with the vital skills and knowledge derived from medical science.

It would also be mistaken, according to Cartwright (1977), to presume that the dissolution of the monasteries at the time of the English Reformation led to a loss of care for the sick and weak. The continental influences on the English Reformation, Lutheranism and particularly Calvinism, envisaged a society in which the sacred pervades the secular (Troeltsch, 1931). This is reflected in Calvin's belief in the Godly magistrate, the Godly state, in which Christian love infused every aspect of day to day life, and was not reserved for those who followed a religious lifestyle that set them apart from their fellow men and women. For Luther, too, this formed the idea of the vocation or 'calling'. Individuals, whatever their station in life, were called to work for God. The community, this collection of inspired individuals working in co-operation, had the task of looking after the weak and sick. Protection and care were the responsibility of the community and took place within it.

We can also argue that when this spiritual inspiration became clouded, so the quality of care deteriorated. This was true in pre-revolutionary France, where Vincent de Paul was horrified by the lack of care for the sick. It was also true in England, where rational and unspiritual religion allowed for inhumane nursing in hospitals as well as the dreadful conditions of the workhouses. Even in our own day we can see the dangers of losing the spiritual dimension that was so fundamental to the development of hospice care. As Aitken, Fuller and Johnson warn, recalling our earlier reference to James and Field (1992) and the bureaucratization of the hospice movement:

> It is particularly important that the spiritual aspect of the hospice movement should be retained. One of the doctor founders of another hospice writes in his annual report: 'The early units had such ideals, but they seem sadly lacking in some newer ones. Without that "extra dimension" we are doing little more than creating yet another specialty. The dead hand of secularization down the years has so often overlooked the springs from which have sprung the essential good.'
> (Aitkin, Fuller and Johnson 1984, p. 154)

The rewriting of nursing history

Nursing has its roots in a tradition of women and also men who bear the fruit of 'the essential good' of care. By example they demonstrated the moral quality of goodness of character which shows them to be 'white underneath'. For them, the difficult and 'menial' tasks of care become a privilege, carried out as the glad duty of service despite their own personal feelings. Such service was neither easy nor comfortable. For Nightingale it involved the terrible hardships of the Crimea; for Agnes Jones, it resulted in death from disease she caught in the Liverpool workhouse. However, this tradition is our heritage, and the influence on nursing as we know it today is immeasurable. We are heirs to a proud legacy.

But is it a legacy of which we *are* proud? Is it even a legacy that we wish to acknowledge? We cannot end this chapter on the historical tradition of care without considering how this inheritance is interpreted by contemporary nursing writers, and so taught to today's nurses. Nursing history taught to nurses in the past proclaimed this tradition, and writers such as Lucy Seymer (1949) and Agnes Pavey (1951) described the story of nursing through the ages as the fruit of faith. However, nursing history taught to nurses today, as for example by Davies (1980), has radically revised this same story of nursing. The question we need to ask is whether contemporary nursing historians have chosen to interpret nursing history in a certain light because of their own convictions.

If we take Powicke's position on historical method we would agree that our purpose in understanding nursing history is to answer the question: 'How can I discover, in the light of the available evidence, what people were thinking?' As Powicke continues:

> . . . it is the first duty of the historian to try to live through the events and to think the thoughts of those who acted them; it starts from the assumption that, although we may never be able to reach it, there is such a thing as historical truth, and it tries to set on one side all the irrelevancies and obstacles which hide the truth from us.
> (Powicke, 1938, p. 9)

Here we enter the complex realms of historiography which we cannot pursue in depth at this point. However, it is broadly the debate about how history is interpreted and whether it is possible for the historian to find objective truth and purpose in history independent of the subjectivity of the historian. This debate formed the essence of the disagreement between Carr (1961) and Elton (1969). Carr held to a specifically Marxist viewpoint and so interpreted the events of history in the light of a definite political purpose. Elton, although agreeing that historians would find purpose in history, objected to Carr's assertion that only his particular interpretation was valid.

For contemporary nursing writers who have sought to rewrite nursing history, current political, sociological and psychological theories have influenced their interpretations. So, for example, Monica Baly's collection of Nightingale's sayings includes very little reference to her religious faith or its effect on her life and work, which as we have seen was fundamental. Baly (1991, p. 2) writes 'In evaluating Miss Nightingale's writings, it is important to see her in her contemporary context', and proceeds to describe her political radicalism, including her views on women's property rights, while totally ignoring the Victorian religious scene, the effects of the religious revival, and the profound influence theology had on her faith and work. Thus Baly ignores one of the most vital aspects of Nightingale's contemporary context, and instead focuses on the weaknesses of her character. We need to ask the question why? Is it because Baly (1991, p. xv) is seeking to minimize the picture of the 'saint' and, as she writes, 'illustrate her patrician point of view and show her fallibility'. However, it should also be asked whether this political interpretation is as unbalanced as the 'eulogy' she is seeking to correct. Is Baly not drawing out an interpretation of Nightingale that fits with her own modern viewpoint? And if so, will this not be reflected in the sayings that she includes in her book? As we have seen, it is a very one-sided and unbalanced interpretation of what was undoubtedly a very complex woman whose influence on modern nursing cannot be minimized. We must conclude that, while claiming to take a Victorian perspective on Nightingale, Baly in fact gives us her own anachronistic judgement.

Baly's modernist, sociological, psychological and political point of view is reflected in similar nursing histories not only of Davies, but also of Abel-Smith (1960), Smith (1982) and White (1978), and has been used by nursing writers such as Salvage (1985), Webb (1986) and Brown *et al.* (1992). The vocational history of care as the fruit of faith is re-interpreted and disparaged according to modern theories and ideologies. Thus, for example, Dingwall and McIntosh (1978, p. 37) suggest that 'the ideology of "vocation", of nursing as a quasi-spiritual calling . . . [involved] elements of self-interest' which offered a return on investment because 'skilled nursing was the principal contribution which medical science could make to recovery from illness'. They argue that this provided cultural legitimation for the employment of unmarriageable middle-class women, which would not threaten the medical division of labour. This analysis, which uses Marxist language, is pure speculation, but it is a dominant theme which has now become accepted and repeated by writers such as Salvage (1985) and Webb (1986).

Similarly, Dingwall *et al.*, referring to Smith's polemical, psychopathological interpretation of Nightingale as narcissistic, express the opinion that

> This may reflect the difficulty twentieth century scholars sometimes have in taking Victorian religious beliefs seriously. In the terms of our own day, it may be better to see her thinking as an attempt to resolve the guilt of a rich liberal intellectual woman who both enjoyed the privileges of her birth and was tormented by the knowledge of the material and spiritual poverty of those whose labour made her position possible.
>
> (Dingwall *et al.*, 1988, p. 37)

Yet, according to eminent historians such as Powicke and Elton, it is bad history to misrepresent the beliefs and motivations of people in history and to rewrite them according to the personal opinion of the historian without examining other possible interpretations. Furthermore, such historical revisions are of more than academic interest, for they inevitably result in misunderstanding of the vocational mindset and its effects on the character of the carer and his or her attitude towards the moral and scientific dimension of care. In this way a new myth is perpetuated.

Thus, for example, Williams' (1978) discussion of the ideologies of nursing (introduced by Dingwall and McIntosh (1978) above) presumes a false and even simplistic dichotomy between the vocation and the profession and thus, inevitably, a misunderstanding of the underpinning philosophy and values. The new myth holds that vocation involves submission and obedience to the medical profession. 'Embodied in an ideology of Vocation, this servile role of nursing and the submission that it required of its incumbents was consolidated and adjusted to psychologically' (Williams, 1978, p. 40). However, the principle of the vocation or calling, on the contrary, involves a primary submission to God, which may and often does involve a radical rejection of and conflict with human authority and the status quo when it fails in its moral leadership. We need look no further than the radicalism of Nightingale, Agnes Jones, Pastor Fliedner, Vincent de Paul, Cicely Saunders and Christ himself, to see the truth of this. The basis of the nurse's calling imposes on her primary moral values that bind her, above all else, to preserving the personhood of the sick person. We must also add, however, that Nightingale and her tradition held authority to embody the ethical. Obedience to authority implied the recognition of moral authority.

Neither is Williams correct in her suggestion that vocation values only the 'menial' unskilled tasks of care which demand obedience rather than independent judgement.

> An ideology of vocation becomes dysfunctional or obsolete where skilled tasks require independent judgement rather than obedience. . . . Since they are not

seen as menial then they do not require a sacrifice of self, but seen as skilled
they require, rather, an assertion of self in creative and innovative action.

(Williams, 1978, p. 41).

We have seen, and cannot overemphasize, that the values of the calling hold
as inextricable the knowledge, skill and technique necessary to monitor
complex machinery and perform difficult clinical procedures, and the vital
tasks of personal bedside care, such as washing, and the cleaning away of
excreta. Both are vital aspects of the relationship of trust.

Towards the future

I began this chapter by suggesting that quality in health care depends on
moral values, and I have examined the values that have traditionally
underpinned quality care. However, with society, as we saw earlier, health
care has moved into a new value system. Here, as MacIntyre (1985) argues,
we have become susceptible to emotivism, the moral position which holds
that values cannot be rationally agreed in the same way as facts, but are
personal expressions of attitudes, preferences and choices. Having cut away
our traditional value system, our new system of liberal individualism offers
us, as we have said, no objective independent position from which to
evaluate moral disagreement. Only personal preference will ultimately help
us to choose between the varying opinions of, for example, a Noddings, a
Dalley or a Blustein.

Furthermore, MacIntyre believes that, in contemporary society, it is the
therapist and bureaucratic manager, by virtue of their imputed skill and
knowledge, whose emotivist values prevail. These values, he argues, are
utilitarian, for ends are given and outside the scope of debate. Both the
manager and the therapist are therefore concerned only with technique, skill,
profit from investment and effectiveness. As MacIntyre (1985, p. 30) writes:
'Neither manager nor therapist, in their roles as manager and therapist, do or
are able to engage in moral debate'. They are uncontested figures, who
engage only in a discourse where rational agreement is possible, the realms
of fact, means and measurable effectiveness.

We are reminded of our earlier analysis of rationalization and
bureaucratization, and we are left wondering whether MacIntyre has
inadvertently described *our* health-care world based on a competitive
business ethic which is unable to speak on human values because it is tied to
a discourse of organizational objectives and sets of prescriptive standards to
meet defined targets. Furthermore, its language of quality is limited to
measurable effectiveness. Is this discourse, which replaces ultimate moral
principles with techniques of productive and psychological effectiveness, a
possible or desirable method for evaluating goodness, the warmth of care
freely given by the human being who is 'white underneath'? Or are we still

implicitly evaluating what makes for effectiveness by the standards of the caring virtues derived from our tradition – assumed but not acknowledged? We live on borrowed time. I suggest that if we are not to lose the humanity and personhood of care we need to acknowledge and relate to our tradition (Bradshaw, 1994). Perhaps then we will be able to build quality in health care for the future.

References

Abel-Smith B (1960) *A History of the Nursing profession.* Heinemann, London.

Aitken J, Fuller H and Johnson D (1984) *The Influence of Christians in Medicine.* Christian Medical Fellowship, London.

Baly M (1991) *As Miss Nightingale Said . . .* Scutari Press, London.

Benner P (1991) The role of experience, narrative and community in skilled ethical comportment. *Advances in Nursing Science* 14, 1–21.

Blustein J (1991) *Care and Commitment.* Oxford University Press, New York.

Bradshaw A (1994) *Lighting the Lamp.* Scutari Press, London.

Brown J, Kitson A and McKnight T (1992) *Challenges in Caring.* Chapman & Hall, London.

Buber M (1958) *I and Thou.* T & T Clark, Edinburgh.

Buber M (1990) Martin Buber. In Kirschenbaum H and Henderson V (eds) *Carl Rogers: Dialogues* pp. 41–63. Constable, London.

Calman K (1993) From the Chief Medical Officer. *Health Trends* 25, 1–2.

Carr E (1961) *What is History?* Penguin, Harmondsworth.

Cartwright F (1977) *A Social History of Medicine.* Longman, London.

Clay RM (1966) *The Mediaeval Hospitals of England.* Frank Cass & Co. Ltd, London.

Constantelos D (1968) *Byzantine Philanthropy and Social Welfare.* Rutgers University Press, New Brunswick.

Cook E (1913) *The Life of Florence Nightingale, Vols 1 and 2.* Macmillan & Co., London.

Dalley G (1988) *Ideologies of Caring.* Macmillan, Basingstoke.

Davies C (ed.) (1980) *Rewriting Nursing History.* Croom Helm, London.

Dingwall R (1977) *The Social Organisation of Health Visitor Training.* Croom Helm, London.

Dingwall R and McIntosh J (eds) (1978) *Readings in the Sociology of Nursing.* Churchill Livingstone, Edinburgh.

Dingwall R, Rafferty AM and Webster C (1988) *An Introduction to the Social History of Nursing.* Routledge, London.

Elton G (1969) *The Practice of History.* Fontana, London.

Enoch M (1967) Afterword: ready for the scrapheap. In Robb B (ed.) *Sans Everything,* pp. 136–40. Thomas Nelson, London.

Gerth HH and Wright Mills C (eds) (1991) *From Max Weber: Essays in Sociology.* Routledge, London.

Harnack A von (1961) *The Mission and Expansion of Christianity in the First Three Centuries.* Harper Torchbooks, New York.

James N and Field D (1992) The routinization of hospice: charisma and bureaucratization. *Social Science and Medicine* 34, 1363–75.

Jarvis P (1996) Commentary on Chapter 12. In Fulford KWM, Ersser S and Hope T (eds) *Essential Practice in Patient-Centred Care*, pp. 193–7. Blackwell Science, Oxford.

Jones AE (1871) *Memorials of Agnes Elizabeth Jones* (ed. by her sister) Strahan & Co., London.

Kosky J (1989) *Mutual Friends*. Weidenfeld & Nicolson, London.

Lanara V (1976) Philosophy of nursing and current nursing problems. *International Nursing Review* 23, 48–54.

MacIntyre A (1985) *After Virtue*. Duckworth, London.

Midgley M (1981) *Heart and Mind*. Methuen, London.

Murdoch I (1993) *Metaphysics as a Guide to Morals*. Penguin, Harmondsworth.

Nietzsche F (1954) *The Portable Nietzsche* (edited and translated by Kaufmann W). Penguin, Harmondsworth.

Nightingale F (1851) *The Institution of Kaiserswerth on the Rhine, for the Practical Training of Deaconesses, under the Direction of the Rev. Pastor Fliedner, Embracing the Support and Care of a Hospital, Infant and Industrial Schools, and a Female Penitentiary*. The Inmates of the London Ragged Colonial Training School, London.

Nightingale F (1882) 'Nurses, training of' and 'Nursing the sick'. In Quain R (ed.) *A Dictionary of Medicine*, pp. 1038–49. Longmans Green & Co., London.

Nightingale F (1888) Letter to the Probationer Nurses in the 'Nightingale Fund' School at St Thomas's Hospital and Nurses who were formally trained there. Original Letters and Prints for Private Circulation held by University College, London.

Noddings N (1984) *Caring: a Feminine Approach to Ethics and Moral Education*. University of California Press, Berkeley.

Pavey A (1951) *The Story of the Growth of Nursing*. Faber & Faber, London.

Powicke F (1938) *History, Freedom and Religion*. Oxford University Press, London.

Quinn E and Prest J (1987) *Dear Miss Nightingale*. Clarendon Press, Oxford.

Robb B (1967) *Sans Everything*. Thomas Nelson, London.

Salvage J (1985) *The Politics of Nursing*. William Heinemann, London.

Saunders C (1986) The modern hospice. In Wald F (ed.) *In Quest of the Spiritual Component of Care for the Terminally Ill*, pp. 41–8. Yale University School of Nursing, Yale.

Seymer L (1949) *A General History of Nursing*. Faber & Faber, London.

Smith F (1982) *Florence Nightingale: Reputation and Power*. Croom Helm, London.

Temple W (1942) *Christianity and the Social Order*. Penguin, London.

Thomas K (1973) *Religion and the Decline of Magic*. Penguin, Harmondsworth.

Titmuss R (1963) *Essays on 'the Welfare State'*. Unwin University Books, London.

Trigg R (1993) *Rationality and Science*. Blackwell, Oxford.

Troeltsch E (1931) *The Social Teaching of the Christian Churches*. George Allen & Unwin, London.

United Kingdom Central Council for Nursing, Midwifery and Health Visiting (1994a) *Professional Conduct – Occasional Report on Standards of Nursing in Nursing Homes*. UKCC, London.

United Kingdom Central Council for Nursing, Midwifery and Health Visiting (1994b) Statement of purpose of the Council; values of the Council. In *Register* No.14, p. 3. UKCC, London.

Walton J (1990) *Method in Medicine*. Harveain Oration 1990, Royal College of Physicians, London.

Warnock G (1988) Kant. In O'Connor D (ed.) *A Critical history of Western Philosophy*, pp. 296–318. The Free Press of Glencoe, New York.

Webb C (1986) *Feminist Practice in Women's Health Care.* John Wiley & Sons, Chichester.

White R (1978) *Social Change and the Development of the Nursing Profession.* Kimpton, London.

Williams K (1978) Ideologies of nursing: their meanings and implications. In Dingwall R and McIntosh J (eds) *Readings in the Sociology of Nursing*, pp. 36–44. Churchill Livingstone, Edinburgh.

Further reading

Bradshaw A (1994) *Lighting the Lamp: the Spiritual Dimension of Nursing Care.* Scutari Press, London.

Cook E (1913) *The Life of Florence Nightingale, Vols 1 and 2.* Macmillan & Co., London.

3

Why care? Ethical and spiritual issues in caring in nursing

Philip Burnard

Nursing and its core manifestation, which is caring, occurs within a certain context. The context of nursing is one of vulnerability and emotional and physical pain. Against this unavoidable inequality of cared for and carer, the question 'why bother to care?' is frequently posed. The other chapters in this book have addressed the ways in which nurses might think about and practise caring. All of this begs an even more fundamental question: why should nurses care? For we can neither take it for granted that they should, nor can we assume that nurses automatically do care. In this chapter, the question of why nurses should care is addressed from various points of view. The chapter concludes with the idea that caring is so much a part of nursing that if nurses do not care, then they are not fully practising as nurses. Before that conclusion is reached, however, the various arguments for caring are explored. The ethical imperative to care is examined, as are the spiritual aspects of caring and the religious motivations to care. This chapter continues the debate introduced by Dr Ann Bradshaw, this time looking more closely at current justification for caring along contractual, ethical and spiritual lines. All people have a spiritual as well as a physical side to their human nature. It is often this spiritual aspect of their person that wisely governs caring attributes and is responsible for the expressed need to care and be compassionate.

Introduction

The previous chapters have addressed aspects related to caring in nursing. We have seen debates about the nature of caring, about the patients' perspectives and about the historical legacy that nursing has inherited. In this chapter I address the following question: *'why should nurses care?'*

Already, the ground is thorny. The question itself begs previous questions. Can we assume that nurses *do* care, as a matter of course? Is caring *necessarily* part of the nurse's role? Are we clear enough about the *nature* of caring to prescribe it as part of that role? For the purposes of this chapter, we must take it as read that caring *is* part of the nurse's role, but that what needs further debate is the *'why'* of the issue. This will not necessarily be a comfortable debate and, as with any 'abstract' debates, more questions will be asked than can ever be answered. If, however, the profession is committed to a critical and reflexive position, then such questions need to be asked.

It would seem that the debate opens up in at least three directions. There would appear to be *contractual*, *ethical* and *spiritual* issues involved. In this chapter, all three will be addressed, although greater emphasis will be given to the last two issues. The contractual issues would seem to be the easiest ones to address.

Contractual issues

In answer to the question *'why should nurses care?'*, we may want to answer *'because they are under contractual obligation to do so'*. We may argue, for instance, that the business of being a nurse involves the notion of caring, and that to offer clients a nursing service is to offer them caring. Not to offer them caring, on the other hand, is not to offer them nursing. In this sense, nursing is *defined* in relation to caring. A possible parallel may be *teaching* and *learning*. It would be odd to argue (as is sometimes the case) that a teacher has *taught* a topic but that no learning took place. To engage in teaching is to engage in the process of ensuring that learning is occurring. If a teacher really has taught something, then students really have learned. If learning has *not* taken place, then a subject has not been taught.

Similarly, we might want to say that if a person is engaged in *nursing*, then they will have *cared*. If they have not cared, then they have been engaged in something, but that 'something' is not nursing. To nurse, then, is to care.

At a more concrete level, it might be argued that care is offered on the basis of patient or client expectation. We might say that the patient or client *expects* care from a nurse as part of the contract that they have entered into. To be a patient, in this case, is to expect care and to be a nurse, in this case, is to offer that care. Similarly, it might be proposed that nurses are *employed* to offer care. Here, the nature of the contract between nurses and employees is based on an expectation that the nurses will offer care. It needs to be said, though, that such a contractual issue is more an *implicit* than an explicit one. It seems likely that very few formal contracts will include 'care clauses' – at least in the short term. It seems possible that, in the future, caring *may* be formalized in this way – and this opens up further problems.

If caring *is* a contractual issue, we need to consider the implications of this. In an important book about caring in the health professions, Campbell

(1984), notes the apparent contradiction of the fact that health professions are called upon to care but are also *paid* to do so. It is as though the health professional is being called upon to 'turn on' their care, according to their financial contract. This state of affairs is similar to that found in counselling and psychotherapy, in which the client pays a professional person to sympathize, empathize and listen. The open question remains: can a person care *professionally* and for money?

The sort of debate that usually occurs at this point is whether or not a paid carer is 'genuine'. The argument seems to revolve around the idea that genuineness is somehow a 'natural' state of affairs, whereas the introduction of a profit motive brings an unnaturalness to the proceedings. This sort of argument often surfaces when people discuss the naturalness or otherwise of cabin crew in aircraft, hotel and restaurant staff and even service staff in McDonald's! A view is often expressed that if people have to be *trained* in working with the public, then they are likely to be 'artificial' or 'unnatural'. This type of argument is sometimes even levelled at a whole country or culture, as is seen in the statement that 'Americans are shallow and insincere'. This sort of sentiment is often based on the high levels of attention paid to greeting and thanking that occur in American service industries. The phrase 'have a nice day' has, for the British, become synonymous with insincerity.

There is, however, another way of looking at all of this. The argument may be levelled that we have *all* 'learned' to relate to others. If we care, we do so because we have *learned* to care. That learning process may have occurred over a number of years. It might be argued, for example, that we learned to care by being cared for – by parents, friends, lovers and partners. We have experienced care and therefore are able to show care in return. We may also have learned to care vicariously – by observing other people being cared for. All of this amounts to a learning process.

If we return to the debate about professional carers, we may find that cabin crew, hotel staff and others have also *learned* to care – but have done so in a highly structured, intentional way. The process has been speeded up and, although the *methods of learning* may be different, it can still be argued that such staff have learned to care. This may also be the case with nurses. There is no reason why we should automatically assume that caring 'comes naturally' to some people, or even that it must always be spontaneous and straight from the heart. There need be nothing particularly sinister about the nurse who sets out to improve her or his caring skills or who plans care for another person. We train counsellors and psychotherapists, and there seems no reason to assume that we should not also train carers. If we can decide upon what constitutes a caring disposition or attitude, then we may be able to isolate the elements that need to be taught in a 'caring syllabus'. At the present time, those elements have *not* been identified particularly clearly, but there is no reason to suppose that future research will not isolate them. Nor need this become a debate over holism versus reductionism. We can analyse the concept of caring – as a means of helping to teach it – without dissecting the *person*. The person remains a 'whole' even if, for training purposes, we filter out some elements of our relationship with that person.

There is another aspect to the *contractual* aspect of caring. Homans (1961) proposed a theory of social exchange. He suggests that:

> The open secret of human exchange is to give to the other person behaviour that is more valuable to him than it is costly to you and to get from him behaviour that is more valuable to you than it is costly to him.

Interpersonal life, for Homans, was a series of transactions in which each person did things for and with another person in anticipation of receiving something. This is a day-to-day example of the general rule that 'there is no such thing as a free lunch'. In this context, it means that nurses care in order to get something in return. They care so that they will be thanked or rewarded in less tangible ways. What reinforces their caring behaviour is the fact of that reward. In this model, no one does things out of empathy or true compassion for others, but by virtue of the fact that there will always be a pay-off. A less cynical view might be that we care *because* we are paid. The 'return', in this case, is payment itself. Either way, the issue of caring is, again, a contractual one. Nurses are employed to be caring and are paid because they care.

There is yet another, more human, aspect to the contractual debate. Martin Buber (1958), in a complicated and meandering essay on interpersonal relationships, compared and contrasted the 'I-It' relationship with the 'I-Thou' relationship. These concepts have slipped into many papers and discussions about the nature of caring. In essence, Buber's argument was this: that when we deal with people on an 'I-It' basis, we turn them into objects. This sort of objectification can be seen when we refer to another person as 'the appendix in bed six'. Suddenly, the breathing, feeling, living person has become 'an appendix' – an object. Buber argues that a more human – and more morally defensible position – is to treat people from the point of view of an 'I-Thou' relationship. In such a relationship, each person meets the other as a conscious, knowing and feeling human being. In meeting you as a 'thou', I respect your humanity. (It should be noted, at this point, that the 'thou' issue is something of a problem in the English language. In the French and German languages – to name but two – 'thou' is the 'familiar' version of addressing another person. In the English language no distinction is made between a 'personal' address and a more 'formal' address, and this makes the discussion of the I-Thou issue a little more complicated because these distinctions are lost.)

What Buber is addressing is another version of the contractual issue (although it shades over into the domain of ethics). He is arguing that part of the process of working with other human beings is to acknowledge *their* humanness. Part of the 'contract' of being a carer or a therapist is *not* to turn them into an object but to allow them to remain people, and people on equal terms with ourselves. To do this involves constant vigilance and a great deal of humility. For if we are to retain the 'I-Thou' mode of relations, we must forego any 'professional' pretensions that we may have, as to treat people from a professional point of view might involve turning them into objects.

These, then, are aspects of the contractual approach to caring. From this point of view, nurse–patient relationships are seen as variously defined and negotiated relationships that involve some sort of give and take on behalf of the two parties. In such relationships, each party is seen as having some type of need that requires fulfilment. Caring, from this point of view, is as much about the fulfilment of various needs as it is an innate human condition.

Ethical issues

Another approach to the question of 'why care?' is an ethical one. Ethical questions concern right or wrong, how to make appropriate decisions, or how to act in a given situation. In this case, we may ask 'on what grounds is it appropriate for me, as a nurse, to act in a caring way?'

There are various ways of approaching ethical issues. One, for example, is through appeal to a religious code of some kind, that instructs the believer in ways to act. As spiritual issues are discussed later in this chapter, those approaches to solving ethical dilemmas will not be addressed here, except to note that most religious codes implore believers to act caringly towards other people. We might even be tempted to argue that a religious person is usually duty bound to act in a caring way towards other people. Ironically, however, even the briefest of glances at the world picture will reveal that religion also underlies many of the international instances of people *not* caring for each other. And therein lies an almost imponderable paradox: that whilst – as far as we can tell – all religions insist on the caring treatment of others, most are also a potential source of very uncaring behaviour.

We need, then, to turn to secular approaches to the ethics of caring. By secular, I mean, in this context, those approaches that do not necessarily draw on religious codes of behaviour – although the two are often compatible. There is no reason to suppose that a secular approach to ethics automatically rules out a particular religious code.

A widely cited source of guidance in ethical matters is Kant's injunction that we should act as though our behaviour was illustrating a universal law of behaviour. In other words, when we act, we must do so believing that the behaviour would be one that *anyone* might reasonably engage in. A right action, then, is one that is *universally* right. This is the basis of Kant's *categorical imperative*.

Using this position, it might thus be possible to argue that the reason we *should* care is that we would hope to be cared for ourselves. We would also hope that care would be extended to all the people that we know and love. In this way, caring is almost a necessary human behaviour because *absence* of care is, by the same token, unacceptable as a universal principle. If I say, for example, that it does not matter whether I care or not, I am (according to the principles outlined so far) arguing that it does not matter whether *anyone* cares. Presumably, I would not want to live in a world in which no one cared for others, and so caring becomes an imperative. Nor does a middle position seem tenable. Presumably, I would find it difficult to argue that it could be a universal principle that people should be 'indifferent' to each other – neither caring nor uncaring. It might even be mooted that such indifference would be *worse* than not caring. The evidence – if it can be called that – from the Kantian principle, seems to be that caring is a necessary human act and one that I am compelled to offer because I, too, am human. To act in less than a caring way is to *justify* a lack of caring.

Another approach to considering ethical issues is Mill's *utilitarianism* – an approach first articulated by Jeremy Bentham. Utilitarianism is often summed up by the slogan that 'that which is good is that which causes the greatest happiness to the greatest number', or slight variants of this. It appears reasonable to argue that caring is *unlikely* to cause widespread unhappiness and, therefore, can be justified as a 'good' action. Put in a positive version, it seems possible to say that it is likely that caring *will* cause fairly widespread happiness, and can again be justified. All this, of course, hangs on how 'caring' might be defined, an issue which has again been the subject of debate throughout this volume. It would seem difficult, however, to argue that caring is *not* a 'positive' concept. Whatever caring is *not*, it seems likely that it can always be defined in positive, life-enhancing ways.

Yet another approach to ethics is via *existentialism*. Existentialism is a particular and distinctive approach to philosophy, and it cannot really be described as a 'school' of philosophy as it is, by its nature, against systems-building, and may even be described as anarchical in its approach. Perhaps the most populist definition of existentialism as an approach to philosophy was offered by Jean-Paul Sartre in his 1949 essay *Existentialism is a Humanism* (usually translated as *Existentialism and Humanism*) (Sartre, 1952). Sartre sums up the heart of existentialism through the slogan 'existence predates essence' and, given existentialism's influence on nursing theory and on patient-centred approaches to care, it may be worth considering it in a little more detail.

What does it mean to say that *existence predates essence?* First, it is often useful to consider the *opposite* of what it means, and the example that Sartre himself cites is useful. He asks the reader to consider a paper knife. Before a paper knife comes into existence, its form and function (or its *essence*) has already been determined. Someone has sat down and given thought to what other people might need to use to open letters. That person has then designed the implement, and other people have worked on manufacturing it. Once the paper knife comes into existence, its 'essence' has largely been fixed.

Sartre argues that, for human beings, exactly the opposite is the case. There is no blueprint for the person. He or she is simply 'thrown into the world' (to borrow an expression from Heidegger). To quote Sartre on this point:

> Man first of all exists, encounters himself and surges up in the world and defines himself afterwards. If man, as the existentialists see him, is not definable, it is because to begin with he is nothing. He will not be anything until later, and then he will be what he makes of himself.
>
> (Sartre, 1952, p. 28)

The existential position, then, is this: that a person 'comes into existence', that that person's 'essence' or 'personhood' only emerges later, and that this essence (and this is a vital point) is whatever that person makes it. He or she is the 'author of his or her essence'. For Sartre, a person is both free and responsible. He or she is free to become whatever he or she makes of him or herself. Because of that freedom, the person is also *responsible* for what he or she becomes. We cannot be free and *not* responsible. Consider, for example, if I make the statement 'I am free to do what I want, but I must check things first with my wife!' Clearly, I am not free. I can *only* be free if I acknowledge that there is no one else that can choose for me. If I am free, I am free to make decisions and those decisions *always* involve the exercise of responsibility. Sartre writes of the 'anguish' of choice. Choosing for oneself is difficult on a number of counts. First, I *must* choose. Even *not* choosing involves a form of 'negative choice'. Secondly, no one, in the end, can make decisions for me – I am on my own. Thirdly, no one can really *advise* me. They have not had my life experiences and cannot take responsibility for the outcome of my life decisions.

If all of this is true for all individuals, it raises questions about how I *should* choose. What rules are there to guide me? Sartre's answer to this is fairly terse, and along the lines of 'there are none!' Choice and decision making, for Sartre, are necessarily lonely and idiosyncratic actions. However, he acknowledges that *everyone* is in this position. I am not choosing in isolation, as I am surrounded by a wide range of 'others' who are also choosing. Thus, when I *do* choose, I nearly always find myself taking into account the effects of those choices on those around me (after all, as we have noted, I carry the responsibility for those choices). Each choice I make is likely to have some sort of impact on other people. Consider, for example, if – as a married person with children – I decide to leave this country and go and live in splendid isolation on a distant island. Clearly, the responsibility for such an action is mine. Only I can decide to do this. However, I must also consider the *responsibility* that goes with such an action. Like it or not, other people will be affected by my action: my wife, my children, my friends, my work colleagues, and so on – there is a ripple effect. This being the case, Sartre suggests that I need to consider this question: 'what would happen if *everyone* acted in this manner?'

At this point, Sartre appears to want to advocate a type of Kantian ethic. Sartre seems to say that we should act as though our action was one that would be *reasonable* for anyone else to carry out. Close reading, though, suggests that Sartre offers a slightly different argument. He suggests that, when I undertake an action, I *must* believe that it is a reasonable action. If I do not, I am deceiving myself: in Sartre's terms, I am acting in 'bad faith'. The 'authentic' person, on the other hand, acknowledges that to choose a course of action *is* to imply that it is a 'right' action and, therefore, one that other people could reasonably be expected to carry out, too. If, for example, I *do* leave my wife and family and live on an island, I am saying something like 'in leaving my family and children and going to live on the island, I am doing a reasonable thing. It follows, then, that I cannot condemn anyone else who does the same thing.' There is a subtle difference, here, between the Kantian ethic and the Sartreian one. Kant is establishing that there are 'universal principles' that determine ethical decisions. Sartre, on the other hand, is suggesting that *individuals* are constantly determining the nature of 'right' actions. In being constantly faced by decisions and choices, people are determining on a dynamic basis what is right and wrong. This is a very 'fluid' view of ethics, and suggests that ethics are situational. I cannot lay down a priori a set of rules or principles for action, because I am still in the process of 'inventing myself'. All I can do is to note that every time I act, I am saying to other people, via my actions, that 'this is a reasonable thing to do'.

All this leads us back to caring. To cut a very long story short, I continue to care because I continue to endorse care as 'right action'. I may not do so tomorrow, and my beliefs and judgements may change as I evolve as a person but, for today, I believe that caring is important. Furthermore, I hope that other people's actions – in so far as they affect me – will also involve caring. I would hope that others would care for me, although I cannot guarantee that they will. Although I cannot even *expect* that they will care, I will continue to hope. In this way, I am also supporting the idea of caring as a positive activity. It is something I would wish *on* other people and *for* other people – at least for the moment.

One of the most liberating – if daunting – features of existentialism is its *dynamic* quality. People, as defined by existentialists, are always in a state of flux: they are always engaged in the process of *becoming*. The human project is never complete. In this sense, we can never define, once and for all, what we *should* or *must* do. All we can do is to continue to review and reaffirm our beliefs – almost on a day-to-day basis. Caring, in this sense, becomes something of an act of faith.

Spiritual issues

As we have noted, a third approach to the question of why we should care lies in the spiritual domain. The whole issue of what 'spirituality' might be referring to is a complex one. While the word itself contains another word, *spirit*, the term has been used more broadly than simply to signify a belief in the inherent *spirit* of a person. However, it is most frequently linked to religion and to religious beliefs.

A distinction needs to be made between the two issues *'spirituality'* and *'religion'*. Religion usually refers to a set of beliefs about a higher being or a transcendental quality. Geertz (1966) bravely attempted to cut through many of the more complex issues surrounding the question of religion by offering the following definition:

> Without further ado, then, a religion is: (1) a system of symbols which acts to (2) establish powerful, pervasive and long-lasting moods and motivations in men by (3) formulating conceptions of a general order of existence and (4) clothing these conceptions with such an aura of factuality that (5) the moods and motivations seem uniquely realistic.

What is important here is that Geertz is noting that religions necessarily hold that their beliefs about the nature of things – even supernatural things – are *true*. This poses something of a paradox. On the one hand, religious beliefs are necessarily just that – beliefs, but on the other hand, the religious person holds those beliefs to be *true*. Thus, for the religious person, *beliefs* have become *truths* – and truths, by definition, are not beliefs but *facts*. It is hardly surprising, therefore, to note the amount of conflict that has occurred between people of different religions, for – presumably – various but different *truths* cannot coexist alongside each other and still remain 'true'. What happens is that each person, if he or she is of an extreme temperament or cultural persuasion, holds *only* his or her set of beliefs to be true and, therefore, all others to be false. Herein lies the source of conflict.

However, there are numerous common elements in different religions. This is not to say that all religions amount to the same thing, or to suggest (as it is popular to do) that all religions have an 'element of truth in them'. Such a notion is as difficult to 'prove' as the tenets of the various religions themselves. It is to note that there are features in most religions that are echoed in most others. One of those issues is the injunction that members of the faith should *care* for one another. In all of the major world religions this idea of caring for one another is paramount. Indeed, it would be difficult to imagine a religion – existent or created – that suggested otherwise. To *care*, therefore, is an essential 'regulation' of religious faiths. It follows, therefore, that the 'religious' nurse is also one who cares, not, interestingly enough, necessarily because he or she is a *nurse* but rather because he or she is a member of that religion or faith.

There is yet another way of looking at this question of caring from a religious perspective. It surrounds the issue of what we might understand when we use the word God. In the 1960s in the field of Christianity there was a considerable debate about the idea of religion without a formal sense of 'God up there or God out there' (Robinson, 1961) – the 'Honest to God' debate. Earlier – and firing this debate – Paul Tillich had described the idea of God in terms of the 'ground of our being', and his definition of God is worth considering at some length because it links so well with this discussion about nursing, religion and caring. Tillich wrote:

> The name of this infinite and inexhaustible depth and ground of all being is *God*. That depth is what the word *God* means. And if that word has not much meaning for you, translate it, and speak of the depths of your life, of the source of your being, or your ultimate concern, of what you take seriously without any reservation. Perhaps, in order to do so, you must forget everything traditional that you have learned about God, perhaps even that word itself. For if you know that God means depth, you know much about him. You cannot then call yourself an atheist or unbeliever. For you cannot think or say: Life has no depth! Life is shallow. Being itself is surface only. If you could say this in complete seriousness, you would be an atheist; but otherwise you are not. He who knows about depth knows about God.
>
> (Tillich, 1949, p. 64)

God, for Tillich, cannot be located 'above' the world, for 'above' can only exist when a 'flat earth' view of the universe is maintained. There can be no easy way of pointing 'up there' from our present view of the universe. To claim that there is an 'up there' would be rather like people in the UK trying to argue that people in Australia are upside down! However, the depth of which Tillich writes is not a depth of some sort of universal geography but a *human* depth: a depth of experience, feeling and being.

If you are to accept Tillich's points about atheism and about knowing God, you must, of course, accept the first point that he makes – about God being 'the same as' depth. He rather seems to assume that the reader *will* make this 'leap of faith'. However, if the reader *does* accept Tillich's view of God, then the idea of *caring* takes on an even more urgent perspective. For the believer who sees God as the 'ground of our being' or in terms of depth is *required* to care for another person simply because that other person *also* contains depth and also has God as the 'ground' of his or her being. It would seem that within Tillich's conception of God is contained the imperative to care for one another, for not to do so is to care less about God.

On a more straightforward level, however, it is possible to note that most religions have a 'code of conduct' – usually written into holy books – that *prescribes* care for others. To care, in this case, is to follow the teachings of that particular religion by reference to its code of conduct. In this sense, the religious view of caring is very much akin to the *moral* view of caring.

But what of the atheist? While Tillich wishes to dismiss atheism or a positive disbelief in the existence of God, others *would* acknowledge that such unbelief is possible. How might the atheist answer the question: 'why should I care?'

He or she might, of course, simply reply 'I don't! I have no reason to!', and that might be the end of the matter. Undoubtedly, for a few people, this is a tenable position and one that is consistent with the notion that there is not an outside force or higher being or ground of our being. However, the fact of being atheist does not *automatically* rule out the necessity to care.

It is interesting to note the position adopted by the *rational humanists* (Blackham, 1961) on this matter. They, as atheists, argue the following position. First, God – as far as they can tell – does not exist. Secondly, because of this fact, we are alone and responsible for what we do. Thirdly, because of *this* fact, we are bound not only to be responsible for ourselves, but also for the whole of mankind. The rational humanist position has something in common with the existentialist position, and much in common with the Kantian imperative. The fact that there is no 'outside arbiter' of what is right or wrong and no one from whom forgiveness can be sought means that we must forge our own morality. We *must* care for each other for *not* to do so is not to acknowledge and respond to the humanity in others. Thus it may be argued that the atheistic position does not exclude the idea of caring for self and others.

There are two other positions that might be considered in this brief review of religious and non-religious positions. They are *agnosticism* and what I wish to call *spiritual neutrality*. The agnostic is the person who believes that, because the existence or otherwise of God can never be proved or disproved, discussion on the matter is irrelevant. We are only ever dealing with matters of *faith* and the question of God can never ultimately be verified. The agnostic, then, is the person who has dismissed religion, consciously, as being beyond debate and argument. More commonly, however, the term is used in an everyday sense to describe a person who is 'not sure': the person who has yet to make up his or her mind about religious matters.

The question of *spiritual neutrality* is a different one. I want to suggest that for a considerable number of people – particularly in the West – the issue of spirituality and religion has little or no relevance. They simply do not weigh up the world and/or humanity in religious or spiritual terms. Religion and spirituality have little or no meaning for them. It is easy, in these days of discussions about 'spiritual needs', to assume that (a) *all* people have spiritual needs of one sort or another – even if these have yet to be identified, and (b) that spiritual matters of one sort or another are, ultimately, important to *everyone*. A common argument amongst those who *do* think about religion and about spiritual issues is that such people have yet to give thought to these issues and that, at some unspecified time, they *will* do so. This becomes an impossible argument, for it is never possible to specify *when* that sort of moment might occur! It seems to me, from the experience of looking after and counselling a range of different people that – for some – spiritual matters, *however those matters are defined* – are irrelevant.

Again, neither of these positions necessarily or logically leads to one of lack of care. It seems quite possible to be an agnostic and to care, or to be spiritually neutral and to care. Indeed (without retreating from the positions outlined so far) it is quite possible to argue that many people will care simply because they choose to do so. Why? Possibly because caring itself is *enjoyable*. In all the rather heavy debate about motives, attitudes, spiritual and non-spiritual issues, it is sometimes possible to lose sight of the sheer pleasure that caring for others can offer, nor need this be a *selfish* pleasure.

I remember, as a child, being impressed by how often my parents would go without certain items in order to pay for things for me. At the time, I imagined that they were incredibly altruistic (although at the time I would not have used that word!). I also thought that they must be martyrs to go without things for themselves in order to provide more for me and my sisters. Now I am a parent of teenage children, however, I appreciate that no heroism or martyrdom is involved. It is simply pleasurable to give to your children. You do not give anything up, you do not think in terms of 'going without', you simply enjoy the giving. I propose that this can also be the motivation behind many acts of caring as a nurse. There *may* be deep-seated religious, cultural or even psychological motives, but there may simply be the straightforward human act of caring that creates pleasure in both the carer and the one who is being cared for.

Summary and conclusions

The answer to the question 'why care?' may come in various forms. We have explored the idea that caring may be a contractual issue. You care because that is what is expected of you and that is what your job consists of. Put less crudely, you care because the essence of nursing is the caring relationship. Not to care is not to be fully involved in doing nursing.

The question has also been tackled from an ethical point of view. It has been suggested that it is possible to argue from a variety of ethical positions that caring is some sort of moral imperative. We care for others because we *must*, or to put it another way, we are able to reflect on our own humanity and we are able to recognize the humanity of others. Once we realize that the world is peopled with creatures like ourselves, we feel (or should feel) the need to treat those 'others' as we would want to be treated ourselves. This issue could, of course, have been opened up in other directions. There have been various *psychological* arguments for the need to treat other people caringly. Freud, for example, posited the idea of a *superego* that 'controlled' our moral actions. Furthermore, he suggested that we 'inherited' our morality from our parents and from the society in which we grew up and that our 'superegos' were largely manifestations of our consciences. We act caringly because not to do so is to invoke a guilty conscience. Living with a guilty conscience may be more difficult than trying to live morally and trying to care for other people.

The question of 'why care?' has also been explored from a spiritual or religious perspective. These two concepts seem inextricably bound up with one another. I have argued, elsewhere, that the concept of 'spirituality' can be broadened to include the needs of atheists and agnostics and that it may not necessarily be linked with religion and with religious experience (Burnard, 1987). I now feel that this is to extend the use of the term so widely as to make it almost meaningless. If the term 'spiritual' contains the word 'spirit', and if the world 'spirit' is linked very closely to religion (of whatever sort) then it seems to me, now, that spirituality and religion cannot be unlinked without stretching the terms almost irreconcilably. In this chapter, I have explored some of the ways in which caring becomes an imperative for the person who has religious beliefs. Often, this imperative comes from a given religion's code of conduct. At other times, though, it comes from beliefs about the nature of God. It also comes from most religions' teachings.

Finally, I have considered the position of caring from the point of view of agnostics and from the viewpoint of those for whom spiritual and religious issues have little meaning. I have suggested that caring can be pleasurable and worthy of pursuit for its own sake. In underlining this position, I would want to add that I am not suggesting the idea of 'pleasurableness' of caring in terms of some sort of 'return', but rather that caring can give unselfish and even 'unrewarded' pleasure.

However it is viewed, it would seem that caring is an almost universal phenomenon and one linked to the very process of becoming and being a person. If that is the case, then caring remains at the centre of the process of nursing for, whatever it is *not*, nursing is intimately bound up with all aspects of the person.

References

Blackham JP (1961) *Humanism*. Pelican, Harmondsworth.

Buber M (1958) *I and Thou*. Scribener, New York.

Burnard P (1987) Spiritual distress and the nursing response: theoretical considerations and counselling skills. *Journal of Advanced Nursing* 12, 377–82.

Campbell A (1984) *Paid to Care?* SPCK, London.

Geertz C (1966) *Anthropological Approaches to Religion*. Tavistock, London.

Homans GC (1961) *Social Behaviour in its Elementary Forms*. Harcourt Brace, New York.

Robinson JAT (1961) *Honest to God*. SCM, London.

Sartre J-P (1952) *Existentialism and Humanism*. Methuen, London.

Tillich P (1949) *Shaking the Foundations*. Pelican, Harmondsworth.

Further reading

Burnard P and Chapman CM (1993) *Professional and Ethical Issues in Nursing: the Code of Professional Conduct*. Scutari, London.

Morrison P (1993) *Professional Caring in Practice*. Avebury, Aldershot.

4

Art and literature: nursing's distant mirror?

Gosia Brykczyńska

As more nurse educators call for the use of humanities in the promotion of caring, it becomes clear that there is little understanding of some of the basic concepts used in the arguments. This chapter therefore looks at some of these concepts, including the nature of aesthetics, the meanings and usage of narratives, and finally the implications of the use of the arts in promoting sensitivity and caring awareness in nursing. There is a paucity of academic literature written by nurses on these subjects, and some of the extant philosophical material can be rather obtuse. If the arts and humanities are to be used in nursing education and practice, and employed to promote a more caring, compassionate attitude among nurses, then it is worth looking more closely at the concepts of beauty, the domain of aesthetics, the significance of narrative and the power and influence of literature, not only to ensure a creative response but also to initiate a deeper appreciation of the wisdom which they contain.

Introduction

Of all the aspects of nursing, the artistic and aesthetic ones are the least commented upon and understood (Darbyshire, 1994a). Either the aesthetic aspect of the work is limited to a form of romanticism, or the artistic side is seen as a form of excellence in the pursuit of competence. Thus, some say, it is the aesthetic side of nursing that portrays the nurse as an angel of mercy and the art-component aspect of nursing that encourages a particular form of bandaging or type of pleasing uniform! In reality, aesthetics, art and the humanities have little to do with any of this.

The humanities are a collection of liberal arts, the main purpose of their pursuit being to broaden one's outlook on human life and the context in which it is lived. The term 'humanities' stems from the endeavours of the early Renaissance scholars, who in an attempt to look at the world in a new way took up the study of Greek and Hebrew in addition to Latin. They studied these subjects in order to be able to examine original biblical texts and read for themselves early Greek and Roman thoughts and literature, in order to be able to understand man, in all of his humanity (Brykczyńska, 1995). Since that time the humanities have taken on a somewhat different presentation. They now consist of the study of the arts, that is, literature, music, painting, architecture, etc., in addition to languages, history, philosophy and theology.

Some authors of nursing have placed great faith in the humanities, which are undoubtedly seen by some nurses as the answer to many of contemporary nursing's problems. The argument they use is that 'compassionate awareness may only develop as a consequence of experience and critical reflection' (Moyle *et al.*, 1995). It is claimed that one of the properties of the humanities is that they are able to deliver vicarious experiences, and provide a mechanism for critical reflection. As Moyle *et al.* (1995) have observed, many nurses do see problems in life, but 'they do not feel particularly troubled by the world in which they exist, except for issues pertaining to current social economic and political events.' However, it is probably doubtful whether the humanities can really promote caring to the extent that these authors claim.

What is probable is that promoting an interest in the arts can widen nurses' perspectives. The arts can specifically help to introduce nurses to ideas, concepts and perspectives which they might not otherwise have been made aware of in the normal course of their own lives. All nurses have personal experiences that help to develop them as individuals, but they often do not have the vocabulary or insights to be able to reflect constructively on them. As Watson (1988) notes, for many nurses the 'human is viewed as greater than, and different from, the sum of his or her parts'. Such approaches to the human individual call for much sensitivity, understanding of psychology and interpersonal communication skills – an observation which Moyle *et al.* (1995) feel that the study of the humanities, especially in the form of literature, can help to advance.

It is my intention to illustrate how the arts, as portrayed in the humanities and as supported by philosophies, endeavour to tell the story of our lives, and thereby help to focus our concerns on the human individual. Our lives are spent in sorrow, pain, everyday greyness, sometimes wariness and even violence. Our professional lives have stories, as do the lives of others. It is the arts, especially literature, that manage so well to portray the narrative of our life, and to demonstrate how an appreciation of this can promote interpersonal caring (Styles and Moccia, 1993). Sometimes historians, writers and artists look specifically at nurses and nurses' stories; Anne Hudson Jones' (1988) work is a lovely example of such a compendium. More recently, Liane Jones (1995) collected together the experiences of twelve nurses over a period of 1 year. Their narratives make compulsive reading. This chapter, however, will predominantly focus on classical and non-professional literature and art and how these typical examples from the humanist arts can promote caring, specifically caring as experienced by nurses.

As Henderson (1991), one of the wisest nurses to have lived commented: 'the nurse who sees herself as reinforcing the patient when he lacks will, knowledge, or strength will make an effort to know him, understand him, "get inside his skin . . ."'. It is a property of art that it helps us get inside other people's skin.

Aesthetics and nursing

Although most people can appreciate the beauty of a summer sunset, the song of a woodland bird or the sheer power and majesty of a stalking tiger, this recognition of beauty in nature does not seem to form an adequate foundation from which to generalize about beauty, and beautiful art in particular. The study of art – the study of what makes something beautiful and artistic and the philosophy that accompanies these thoughts, is called aesthetics. Since nurses are increasingly looking to the arts to promote a sensitivity towards caring, it is appropriate that we understand what is meant by art and what is meant by aesthetics (Watson, 1993/94).

Many philosophers have commented on the nature of art and the philosophy of art, and some philosophers have either been known to be very interested in the question of art, or have been considered to be very sensitive and artistic themselves. Jonathan Ree, in a wonderful exposé of thoughts surrounding these issues in a collection of essays looking at the interrelationship of philosophy and literature, notes that some philosophers not only wrote on the subject of aesthetics but were considered to be quite literary and poetic themselves, e.g. Plato, Descartes and, in more modern times, Hegel and Heidegger (Ree, 1987). The reason why philosophers are so interested in the arts and what makes a mere object into a piece of art – the focus of admiration and fascination, is that the arts, and beautiful things, sounds, words and pictures, mean so much to us.

It is the centrality of the arts in our lives that compels the philosopher to scrutinize this object of our fascination. However, philosophers are not so much concerned with the content of art, that is, with the subject matter itself, although where social psychology and philosophy overlap, and where these two subject areas impinge on ethics, they would be more inclined to have a natural interest. Philosophers in general, though, are mostly interested in the nature, or essence, of art. They are interested in the essence of what makes a painting or a book, or a piece of music, a piece of art – that is, something beautiful and aesthetically pleasing. Certainly there are many ways of appreciating art and therefore of commenting on it, but one of the fundamental questions which we must pose before we proceed is the question 'why bother at all?'

Why bother to ask 'what is art?', and 'why bother with art at all?' These two related questions need to be posed because that which we call art, specifically beautiful art, can have such a profound effect on us and can influence our lives so profoundly. The often quoted lines about Helen of Troy, that her face launched a thousand ships, illustrate not so much the poetic licence of the Homeric ballad, as the accepted folk wisdom that beauty can profoundly affect us, and that we can go to great lengths to protect, obtain and promote that which we admire and in which we find pleasure. We therefore need to know what this thing which we call art actually is, and where appreciation of beauty and art fit into our daily lives – lives which we try to give meaning to, lives which we try so assiduously to beautify, and lives that also have a wonderful tale to be told and enacted. Lives that as nurses we are constantly intruding into, often changing, and sometimes closing.

There are several classic arguments as to why we should bother about art, such as its centrality in our lives, its power to convey ideas, the sheer enjoyment and pleasure it provides, and its ability to reflect the world around us, to name but a few. Concerning the last argument, however, we need to be mindful of the retort, articulated by Arthur Danto (1981), that perhaps we do not need to bother ourselves with 'detached images of the sun, the stars and the rest, when we can see these things already, and since nothing appears in the mirror which is not already there in the world to be seen without it' (Danto, 1981, p. 9).

This argument, which was brought forward and articulated by Danto, examines the premise that in fact we not only look at the stars and the sun and the wheatfields, but actually already see what there is to be seen artistically. It would appear, however, that not everyone is capable of such unaided 'vision' of the artistic world around them. The artist Van Gogh looked at the stars like many before him and since, but in addition he 'saw' the motion of the stars, the fluid depth of the Milky Way, the poetry and activity of an otherwise 'fixed' firmament. There is no doubt that I cannot 'see' or paint starry nights over southern France – yet his perception of those ink-black nights, studded with bright lemon-yellow stars set in whirling circles of ultramarine and even shades of green, have permanently altered the way in which I now see starry nights, often in far away places, myself. The power of his art has, to use the language of Danto, transfigured the commonplace into something wonderful and above all memorable (Danto, 1981). It is now difficult for me to tell whether I see starry nights in the light of Van Gogh's paintings, or whether Van Gogh's paintings have permanently influenced the way I see, and above all perceive, starry nights. This phenomenon can also occur with literature, especially poetry.

The 'mirror' argument is one of the more important ones which we attach to the arts, and is fairly persuasive. However, artists can only show us, tell us and compel us to hear, see or appreciate what is already in our psyche. It is there all the time, and around us from the first days of our existence. It is the artist's unique talent, though, often unrepeatable and incomprehensible to us, that facilitates for the rest of us a far better understanding of and a better mastering of the world around us and within us. There is, of course, the danger that we can, metaphorically, fall in love with the image instead of the real thing. To this argument one would have to add that sometimes we can find the image beautiful and compelling but would have no intention of 'desiring the real thing'. For example, a beautiful Stubbs horse can be appreciated for its equine qualities transposed on to canvas, but this does not imply that we need to appreciate real horses, or would desire to ride them or even own them.

Perhaps the real problem with the mirror argument is that whereas we have no choice regarding what surrounds us and forms the fabric of our lives, and therefore must make moral assessments about the significance of what we see, hear, are touched by, etc., there is the potential in art, which mirrors reality, to distance the viewer inappropriately from that which is portrayed. This problem of the suitability of life and all its trappings as the subject of art has provoked much intense debate. Put another way, the question posed is 'Can art in all its various forms reflect all of life, in all its various guises?' Some artists feel that art is above such deliberations – that all of life and its realities are the legitimate subject of discussion, portrayal or presentation. Other members of society, and indeed some artists, feel that some subjects that pertain to the narrative of our life, and indeed which are very relevant to our lives, are not appropriate subjects for artistic portrayal or presentation.

As Danto comments, 'it would be wrong or inhuman to take an aesthetic attitude, to put at physical distance certain realities' (Danto, 1981, p. 22). The problem with representing or mirroring the world around us, even in the context of art, is that it is taking the commonplace and making out of it an artistic statement, i.e. a distancing and objectifying statement about something – yet the critics say some things should not be distanced or objectified. They are considered too intimate, too personal or, as Danto (1981) concludes, 'there are things it would be almost immoral to represent in art, precisely because they are then put at a distance which is exactly wrong from a moral perspective.'

The kinds of 'things' one has in mind invariably concern the pivotal moments of our lives – those aspects of the story of our life that are so powerful and personal that we have to be very careful how and when they are recounted, and how and when they are re-enacted. It is not so much a moral taboo that stops us from portraying certain aspects of our lives artistically, as the realization that, however awe-inspiring, or full of wonder, or powerful a particular story 'may be, by objectifying it, and making it' the subject of Art, we commit the moral crime of distancing ourselves from that which is, by its very definition, intimate, personal and involving.

Some time ago, the arts critics of the serious press were appalled by the decision of an art gallery to allow a young jewellery designer to display earrings, each of which consisted of a tiny 1-inch-long fetus. The critics concluded that the human fetus was not appropriate subject matter for art, even though it can be awe-inspiring, and certainly, paradoxically, the adult nude was deemed to be an appropriate subject matter for Art. The art critics felt that the ultimate objectification of the human being (and surely the whole fascination with the human fetus is that it is an immature human being) made it an inappropriate subject for Art. We can likewise think of the inappropriateness of painting patients dying in a hospice, as if the necessary distancing required to produce the painting in some way confirms the necessary objectification of the subject, i.e. terminal care and the patients who were dying. This form of objectification of one of life's most intimate moments is considered by some to be an inappropriate subject for an artistic painting. However, this consideration stands in opposition to sensitive paintings, for example, of patients in a hospital, even in a cancer department – witness the recent, fairly well-received exhibition of paintings at the Barbican Centre in London by Susan MacFarlane, portraying women receiving treatment for breast cancer (Patrick, 1995). Finally, when artists take artistic photographs, or keep photographic chronicles of pivotal events such as wars, deaths, or natural disasters, the same questions can and often are raised. Even if the photographs are truly artistic, or the subject matter is truly common to and representative of daily toil and pain, the question can be posed, should it be portrayed as art, and is it indeed artistic? Do outsiders, by looking in and commenting on the artistic merits of the form and structure, thereby also distance themselves from the painful subject and content of the photographs? It can also be argued that sensitive photographs can promote a caring disposition (Darbyshire, 1994b).

   In recent years, a chronicle of the last months and weeks of the life of a Midwestern farmer has been published by his surviving family members, and the collection of photographs and commentaries about these final moments of the man's life has been made public (Jury and Jury, 1976). It is hard to know whether this can be considered as art; certainly some of the photographs are artistically made, and the collection of photographic material demonstrates much insight and sensitivity. The question raised by Danto (1981) remains, however, whether or not some aspects of our lives are not none the less considered to be outside the domain of Art. Sometimes we can profitably record the world around us, and it coincidentally happens to be an artistic endeavour, but this is not the art that Danto (1981) or Sheppard (1987) have in mind when they are referring to the subject matter of Art. It is perhaps of interest to note here that these deliberations seem to focus predominantly on the visual arts and possibly drama/film, but they do not appear to focus so much on music or the written word. When a particular story is narrated, the teller of the tale *is* considered to be sufficiently involved with the subject matter to exclude accusations of 'distancing', even when he or she is supposedly only 'reporting' as a disinterested third party. This has several interesting implications for nurses and nursing practice, as the use of literature to promote caring attitudes is becoming commonplace, and personal narrative is used to promote nursing arts almost indiscriminately in nursing education (Leininger and Watson, 1990; Styles and Moccia, 1993; Watson, 1993/1994).

The artistic narrative

The artistic and psychological involvement of the 'writer' in the narration of tales is well documented. In recent years there has been much interest in the social and psychological function of oral history, and the artistic merit of 'the narrative' in many different disciplines, from theology to literature and, recently, nursing (Hudson Jones, 1988; Downie, 1994; Zalumas, 1995). Anthropologists and theologians have for many years analysed the significance of 'the narrative' for its cultural import and psychological and spiritual function. As the famous French linguist and literary critic, Ronald Barthes, has noted, 'narrative is present in every age, in every place, in every society; it begins with the very history of mankind, and there nowhere is nor has been a people without narrative' (Barthes, 1977, p. 79). In anthropological terms we might talk of myth, but of course not all narrative is myth, even if it fulfils basic primordial, culturally relevant functions for a particular society. As Barthes adds, 'All classes, all human groups, have their narratives, enjoyment of which is very often shared by men with different, even opposing, cultural backgrounds' (Barthes, 1977, p. 79).

When narrative becomes accepted folk wisdom, or when it begins and continues to reflect group-accepted stereotypes and norms, it may become 'a myth'. Myths of course are of enormous importance, for in the telling and re-telling of the mythical tale, 'truths' are confirmed, ideas conveyed, history re-lived, retold and re-affirmed, and above all, 'the world is put to rights'. As Marina Warner commented in her series of Reith Lectures in 1994, on the subject of myths, 'Stories held in common, make and remake the world we inhabit' (Warner, 1994, p. 93). Nursing, like other groups, also has its collective narratives. Myths in nursing abound and, like the function of all myths in societies, shape and re-affirm nursing identity, by reaching back to the past to gaze dimly at nursing's glory. As Warner notes, 'The struggle for the story of the past sets markers on the map of the present, which in turn chart the future' (Warner, 1994, p. 85). However, it is almost fashionable these days to disempower myths, to break up traditional tales and to rewrite 'accepted' history, and this tendency also holds true within nursing. Whereas it is true that some myths are 'unreasonable', or are now serving as faulty methods of adjustment to a current situation, for example, the myth that in the past nursing was more rewarding and less stressful – and stories are brought forth to support this claim – not all myths are of this nature. Such myths probably do not serve a very useful purpose, but the wholesale destruction of all myths and legends is shortsighted and spiritually devastating. People need stories, even very fanciful stories. Myths, legends and narratives serve the necessary function of re-affirming cultural truths and identity, for example, that nurses *do care*, and even when the truth of the matter is questionable, the story – the myth that is being told, is attempting to say how it ought to be. There is an element of the ideal in myths. By elevating to perfection the past, a message is sent out as to how we should function and view the present world, at the present time. To this extent Radsma's (1994) article, which queries the assumptions that nurses do care and are 'about caring', misses an important psychological point. It is part of nursing's narrative, embedded in myth, that nursing is about caring, and 'real' evidence that this is not necessarily so does not alter the power and function of the myth, or even bring into question its origin. To query the myth about caring is indeed to query the basic function of nursing. This can be an important and necessary task, but one which, I would argue, is independent of presumed reality. We query the nature of nursing in order to nurse *even better*, not to abolish nursing myths, which have a similar aim!

There is of course the problem of memory. In narrative, memory is not only selective, but also creative. As Warner comments, 'memory leads down many roads' (Warner, 1994, p. 85), and revived memories tell not only the story at hand but, with the benefit of hindsight, put that story into context. The 'Roads of Memory' show where the intersections are to be placed, where major arteries have been built and where they *now* all lead. In the process of building up the myth, narrative is used creatively and memory is selective – for a picture needs to be painted that depicts a *specific* story. Thus Warner concludes that certain memories fall into certain cultural patterns. In addition, the myth needs to take on a particular format and thus, using the classic example of the myth of 'home', she notes, 'Home takes us back to a golden afternoon in the past, and this brings in the question of memory, which in turn raises history as an issue' (Warner, 1994, p. 84). Obviously not everyone has the memory of 'home' as 'a golden afternoon', but the myth tends to depict the feeling of home as a distant carefree memory of 'a golden afternoon'. In desperately trying to tell the story of 'home', mythical 'home' needs to be grounded in an acceptable reality which includes securing it to a place. Home is not only a concept of time, it is also a concept of place, thus 'At the core of the struggle for home lies the struggle for the way the story of place is told' (Warner, 1994, p. 86). How we describe this place 'is where our creative and selective' memory comes in.

It is interesting that only certain people are sanctioned to tell certain tales; only certain people can really 'know' what it *was* like, or what it *is* like. There is a certain common understanding that the myth or legend needs to be part of one's own personal history, or part of the history of one's people, society or profession. Alternatively, if one has 'studied' the myth sufficiently and completed an appropriate apprenticeship, this in turn entitles one to tell the tale. We see this occurring among historians who are not nurses, but who write nursing histories, or among authors who are not themselves privy to pain and suffering or to the world of health care, when we 'allow' them to narrate the tale. However, there are some tales that only the initiated can tell, and these are usually the tales of unspeakable suffering, e.g. stories about life for Jews in concentration camps. Some purists say that outsiders are in a better position to get the story right, and that they see things more objectively, but this is not the point. With myths and legends, it is not objective truth that is being re-told, but a selective, creative reinterpretation of a lived-through memory. The story is personal, biased and inaccurate, but it tells an important tale as perceived by the narrator and, to that extent, is totally unique and yet potentially and simultaneously totally universal. As Warner concludes, 'Even while stories are patently connected to particular places and peoples, as in the case of Hindu epics or Irish legends, they are not immutable' (Warner, 1994, p. 88). Even personal tales can be understood and 'adopted' by third parties – by those who in deliberate attentiveness see themselves in the mirror of time's legend – because as Warner continues, 'They are not even recoupable in some imagined integrity, because the act of recuperation itself and the context of the retelling affect the interpretation' (Warner, 1994, p. 88). The context wherein the story is told is as important as the acts of listening to it and reacting to it – it is a living and dynamic process.

Ronald Barthes (1977) has a few more relevant observations to make concerning the power, function and structure of narratives. As noted with regard to the function of myths, the historical validity of myths is secondary to the importance of their very existence. Likewise, literary merit, although significant, is not the main issue in the analysis of narratives. Barthes puts it rather bluntly when he notes that 'Caring nothing for the division between good and bad literature, narrative is international, transhistorical, transcultural: it is simply there, like life itself (Barthes, 1977, p. 77). It is this aspect of narrative that interests us most. The universal use of narrative and the need for myth and story telling is what interests nurses who themselves have stories to tell, form part of the fabric of the stories that others tell, and who listen creatively to stories that patients relate about their lives. Narratives reflect the process of living as much as they strive to give meaning to living, as Barthes concludes, 'Narrativism can only receive its meaning from the world which makes use of it' (Barthes, 1977, p. 124). To the extent that nurses give narratives a meaning, they are also able to make creative use of them.

Finally, the very linguistic structure of narratives is interesting. Barthes claims that little is known about the origin of narratives, but that the history of narrative can reasonably be assumed to be contemporaneous with that of monologue: 'a creation seemingly posterior to that of dialogue' (Barthes, 1977, p. 124). This seems plausible in that first one 'talks' to oneself, then one talks to anyone who will listen, and finally one is ready to listen to others and respond to their stories. At that point dialogue is born. This observation has a secondary and more serious implication in that, if one cannot find the thoughts and words to 'talk to oneself', then certain truths are not articulated, even to oneself, and although the lived experiences are there, they are not being formulated, analysed or creatively structured. Such a predicament for an individual precludes the possibility of subsequent dialogue. Obviously such people can tell their tales in other ways, in other art forms, via other creative outlets or, if all else fails, they can rely on the artist to express their monologue, their story, for them. It is a form of vicarious personal narration that is commonly adopted and used in our society. To force individuals to tell their own tale in their own words can be rather presumptive and very intrusive.

In nursing, there is currently a fashion to ask students to reflect on practice, and to keep their own journals about their experiences in nursing. Whereas some nurses will find this an interesting and creative exercise, for others it will be an excruciatingly intrusive and anxiety-provoking process, especially if it is linked to some form of assessment. We all have experiences from which a story will and can be told, but not all narratives are verbal. Furthermore, the essence of 'narration' is that it is a prose-poem told because there is something that needs to be told. Moreover, the prose-poem is personal and often 'unshareable'. If, on the other hand, there is nothing that needs to be recounted, or if there is a lack of words to encapsulate the experience, then there is no story to be told, at that time. At the risk of sounding global, and falling into the trap of generalities, most great stories are recounted with the benefit of maturity and the passage of time. For each of us, our meaningful stories are personal and often need to lie dormant for the necessary reflection to take place. Great stories that become the core of epics are usually told after the passing of time; they age like good wine, having lain dormant, maturing slowly in the furthest nooks of our memories of lived experience. When the time is ripe we descend into these dusty cellars and retrieve the memories. They are by then respectfully aged, ready to be shared and, needless to say, creatively interpreted, biased and with a particular focus of attention. We now have something to say! To speed up this process, or even to force it upon someone is of doubtful benefit, and certainly can be very damaging to the psyche.

Poets have often used the ploy of narrative to tell the epic tale. From the unsurpassed depths of Homer's *Odyssey* to the European epic ballads such as the *Song of Roland* or the *Ballad of the Battle of Igorove*, or the haunting Gaelic ballads recounting a people's history, the timing of the stories and the reason why they are retold is quite revealing. There can also be stories within stories, such as Chaucer's *Canterbury Tales*, Bocaccio's *The Decameron*, and so on, written as literary devices to give opportunity for tales to be aired.

This ancient strategy neatly introduces the issue of who the narrator actually is. Who actually owns the tale? In personal narratives, such as the story told by patients of their own life, for the most part the narrator is the person who is telling the story and who is also the subject of the story, although even here there will be moments when some comments made by the narrator will be 'borrowed' from others. They will be telling us the tale from their own perspective as a participant and from the perspective of an outsider, e.g. as themselves, but also as one who is 'a father' – a role description imposed on them by virtue of a specific relationship. However, the questions which philosophers and society pose are, especially when the narrative is in the written form, who is actually telling the tale, who is responsible for the content, and whose story is it? As Barthes (1977) observes, 'who speaks (in the narrative) is not who writes (in real life) and who writes is not who is.' These observations are of crucial importance when analysing narratives in literature and art, for the temptation to accuse the singer of singing an unpleasant song is very strong. The writer of a tale is not the 'person' who also happens to write, and the subject matter of their writing in narrative form does not necessarily represent how they as people (who happen to write) actually feel about the story. It is this latter aspect of narrative that sometimes appears to be forgotten in nursing circles.

It is thus the genius of artists that they can become 'another', sing someone else's song, tell someone else's story, or paint someone else's picture. They do this so well that we indeed confuse the messenger with the message. We assume that the story belongs to them personally, despite the fact that, at the same time, we feel it is our story! It is one of the marks of greatness that an artist can conceive of something to some extent alien to them, or in some instances totally imaginary. It is the American New England poet Emily Dickinson who so succinctly put it, stating:

> I never saw a moor,
> I never saw the sea;
> Yet know I how the heather looks,
> And what a wave must be.

> (Dickinson, 1960, p. 99)

Artists imagine what it must be like to be ill, in pain, poor, or physically or mentally broken, and in telling the tale, take on the persona and language of the characters who they are describing. They become the characters' narrator. The greater the literary artist, the better the quality of narrative, such that the insights and narratives of Shakespeare's characters have become universal, even though Shakespeare himself lived in sixteenth-century England and was very closely bound up with the culture of his time.

Needless to say, should an artist, writer or painter himself or herself go through the horror, joys, exhilaration or sadness which they are depicting or striving to recount, to that extent the narrative usually becomes much more intense and personal and, for the person reading the narrative or looking at the picture, that much more authentic. Goya's paintings of the Franco-Spanish War carry an awesome weight, as do Picasso's images of the destruction of the Basque country, crystallized in his epic painting *Guernica*, now hanging in the Prado, Madrid. Likewise, paintings smuggled out of prisons or concentration camps, despite their often insignificant artistic merit, carry a weight of authenticity that a formal 'court painter' could never hope to achieve. Here it is the authenticity of the narrative that is so important.

In literature, we often acknowledge the depth of perception that accompanies the writer who has also, coincidentally, 'been there'. Thus Alexander Solzhenitsyn's epic narrative *Cancer Ward* undoubtedly rings as true as it does because the author himself spent some time in an oncology unit. This obvious credibility issue can only be taken so far; Solzhenitsyn does not overtly identify himself with Kostiaglokov, any more than Evelyn Waugh saw himself reflected in the jolly characters of *Vile Bodies*, not to mention in the person of Sebastian in *Brideshead Revisited*. None the less, it is in the very nature of a genius to tell someone else's tale and to do this so convincingly that we lose sight of the literary imposition.

It is therefore of great professional interest to us when someone has a poignant tale to tell and also has the genius of narration. This occurs quite often, but it is of course unpredictable and a terrible paradox. The very depth of authenticity becomes the harrowing backdrop to a poignant narrative, such as the parents' tales in the collection of parents' narratives presented by Cooper and Harpin (1991), or the recently edited and presented nurses' 'tales' collected by Liane Jones (1995). Authenticity and credibility can of course come at a very high price, and neither is it that obvious that just because one has something important to say, one will automatically have sufficient insight to know how to recount one's tale, or be able to pass from the monologue phase to dialogue. Perhaps what the artist does so well is to present someone else's tale for interpretation and, as a criterion of greatness, engage us in a dialogue. We become different people, think new thoughts and revise previously held notions precisely because we have entered someone else's narrative and become involved in their dialogue. It is this quality of narrative that makes it so useful a tool in nursing and why, in promoting the humanities, especially literature, we look so closely at the stories that are being told in all their various forms, and try to learn to listen to the contemporary stories of our peers. The purpose of listening to the stories of our peers is not to indulge in literary psychological voyeurism, but to be able eventually to engage in dialogue – creative, curative and caring dialogue.

Nursing and literature

Nursing is about the care of, care for, and care in cooperation with people, usually in times of physical, mental or spiritual distress, discord or deficit. Any artistic form that can capture the ordinariness of this life and its vagaries, and therefore the ordinariness of nursing as it impinges on this life, should therefore be of interest to nurses.

Beverley Taylor, examining the human relationship that nursing represents in an interesting study on the 'ordinariness of nursing', comments that, 'Essentially, being human is about living in the world of other people and things' (Taylor, 1994, p. 3). It is precisely because being human involves the living out of 'stories' in other people's scripts that it is interesting to see what literature can tell us about living, lives spent and events retold, and interrelationships and how we react to them. As Taylor continues, 'If nurses begin to appreciate their potential for understanding interpersonal relationships, they may come to understand themselves as humans who share commonalities with the people in their care' (Taylor, 1994, p. 3). It is one of the main characteristics of literature that it verbalizes events in and aspects of our lives such that the reader can see and appreciate, as Taylor notes, 'themselves as humans who share commonalities with the people in their care'.

There are of course many forms of literature, and one form that seems to be both universal and timeless, and one of the first that we are introduced to as children and often return to as adults, is the so-called fairy-tale. At some level, fairy-tales are forms of myths and legends; at another level, they are the first form of literature that many children are introduced to in our Western culture. Through fairy-tales and children's stories, the immature, developing young person comes to grips with the world around him or her, and the adult finds reassurance and cultural stability.

It is Bruno Bettelheim, the sensitive and versatile child psychologist, man-of-letters and homespun philosopher who, in his extremely accessible book on the nature, function and significance of fairy-tales, notes that the intrinsic message of fairy-tales is that 'a struggle against severe difficulties in life is unavoidable, (it) is an intrinsic part of human existence. . . .' (Bettelheim, 1976, p. 8). This message is seen in the classic stories of *Hansel and Gretel*, *Sleeping Beauty* and *Little Red Riding Hood*, with more contemporary versions of the same message encapsulated in the stories of Hans Christian Anderson, e.g. *The Ugly Duckling*. What traditional fairy-stories have in common is a plain story-line that, in its obviousness, blatantly demonstrates that life is difficult. In the comfort and security of a child's home, these truths can be explored and anxieties reduced. Some fairy-stories, because of the language and metaphors which they employ, can seem either inappropriate in our age or, in today's moral and social climate, need to be rephrased. None the less, the basic idea which they encapsulate is that life is not only hard, but even unjust and cruel, a form of reality confirmation that many modern psychologists would find quite acceptable. The trick, they would argue, is to explain to the child how to overcome this, what to do next. As Bettelheim continues, despite the harshness and cruelty of life, 'if one does not shy away but steadfastly meets unexpected and often unjust hardships, one masters all obstacles and at the end emerges victorious' (Bettelheim, 1976, p. 8). It is this tendency for things to turn out all right, for the 'good guys' to win, for the Princess to find her Prince Charming, that softens the reality contained in the body of the story.

The fairy-story, with its monsters, 'baddies' and gremlins, and in modern versions, plainly naughty children, help the child to adjust to his or her own realities and the reality of the world around him or her. As Bettelheim observes, 'Children know that they are not always good; and often, even when they are, they would prefer not to be. This contradicts what they are told by their parents, and therefore makes the child a monster in his own eyes' (Bettelheim, 1976, p. 7). This 'monster' needs to be understood, tamed and, if necessary, banished or at least controlled. It is one of the functions of fairy-tales and children's stories that they help the child to process some of the problems of growing up and having to form relationships with the world around him or her. Many modern stories for children accomplish this extremely well. They are, for both the child and the adult, perennial favourites, and it is not particularly surprising that the common ingredients, in modern tales as well as in classic fairy-tales, are a story-line containing a lived, understood, identifiable truth, charming, whimsical and often quite intricate illustrations, and beautiful writing. As Bettelheim notes, 'The fairy-tale could not have its psychological impact on the child were it not first and foremost a work of art' (Bettelheim, 1976, p. 12).

It is this artistic link, which we shall encounter again and again, that prompts us to look so closely at the humanities and what they have to offer in terms of our moral and spiritual development. It is precisely because a story is beautifully written and beautifully presented that it becomes memorable. It is not *only* the story-line that is significant in fairy-tales; as some contemporary psychologists contend, such tales may even be too brutal and frightening, but above all it is the packaging. It is the language and drawings that accompany the stories that give them their artistic qualities. Obviously, great art is never, by definition, trivial. It is the property of these stories that they take the everyday, ordinary and mundane and transpose it, on to another distant (and therefore safer) plane. With these fables and tales the child can start to learn not only to appreciate the world he or she is living in, but also to appreciate beautiful entities – beautiful language, beautiful pictures. All of this takes time, and the memorable qualities of these stories facilitate the processing of the child's anxieties and fears.

The recalled story can help the child to understand his or her world, often at a considerably later date. Although adults also help to interpret the world for the child, at a most basic level, children have to think through on their own the significance of life events that take place around them. As Bettelheim concludes, 'We grow, we find meaning in life, and security in ourselves by having understood and solved personal problems on our own, not having them explained to us by others' (Bettelheim, 1976, p. 19). The more artistic and memorable the story, the more likely it is to be recalled and, indeed, consigned to memory, ready to help us to understand life and its events at some later date. It is therefore all the more surprising that, whereas we are prepared to accept the rationale for presenting children with beautiful stories, both classic and modern, in order to help them understand their (and also our) world, this logic seems to end with late childhood. We apparently no longer see the need to encourage even adolescents and certainly not adults to take up a good, well-written book to help them interpret the world, and sometimes to help them tame it.

This is not entirely true, of course, and the sheer variety of 'stories' and written material are testimony to the enduring artistic qualities of narratives, but also testimony to society's need to read, and in so doing process the realities of life. This need would appear to be universal. The Japanese novelist, Naka Kansuke (1976), in a collection of autobiographical short stories, tells of the day on which his teacher, after much prompting, decided to recount the story relevant to a picture hanging on the wall in the classroom. As the novelist commented, 'the most popular lesson was Ethics, because our teacher told us interesting stories about the pretty pictures hanging on the wall.' This form of 'moral development', utilizing narrative with or without visual props, is well known and certainly, as evidenced in this case, not specific to European culture. The problem with this approach, of course, is that the stories, their content and interpretation can be selected, biased and fashioned to suit the specific needs of society and the adult world. This has also been well documented in many cultures, e.g. Soviet Russia, Colonialist England, and so on, and probably is to some extent unavoidable. However, the child may or may not hear the narrative in the same way as the adult. When one chooses to find a different meaning in a story to the accepted version, shame, derision or simply incredulity may ensue. Thus young Naka Kansuke found the story (about the slaughter of Europeans by Japanese during the Japanese War of 1940–45) moving and culturally haunting. However, his teacher commented: 'Not interesting, was it? When I shook my head in protest, he looked surprised and all the children giggled contemptuously.' In the process of reading literature and interpreting literature, whether one is working with children or adults, there must always be sufficient room for novel understanding and different interpretations.

In one of the short stories written by Oscar Wilde for children, *The Devoted Friend*, the more than obvious moral message and social lesson contained within it, that would surely make La Fontaine blush, encapsulated several important points. In the safety of analogy and allegorical concepts, the animals in the story re-enact the age old problem of trust, commitment and the value of friendship. As the Linnet, who is telling the story, comments at the end of the fable to the Duck, who is listening in, 'I have told him a story with a moral.' 'Ah! That is always a very dangerous thing to do,' says the Duck (Wilde, 1888, p. 92). Stories, with obvious moral messages may be difficult to accept, but are stories with hidden messages any more acceptable, and is it a function of literature not only to tell a story, but also to contain a moral?

Stories, that is narratives, can be told and read on any number of levels, and even the most simple and mundane of stories can have a depth to it that is out of proportion to its actual content. This, of course, is what, among other things, differentiates the average story from a piece of great literature or, at any rate, enduring literature. It is also a characteristic of good literature that not only does it survive the test of time, at least to some extent, but also it appeals to more than one generation at a time. This occurs in the classic narrative stories of childhood, such as *Alice in Wonderland* or *Wind in the Willows*, *Winnie the Pooh* or *Huckleberry Finn*. These classics of Anglo-Saxon children's literature all share an inter-generational appeal; indeed some of them, such as *Alice in Wonderland*, contain several cleverly disguised plots running simultaneously, some for children, and some for adults.

Benjamin Hoff, in a book looking at the wisdom contained in *Winnie the Pooh*, notes that at one level the story can be considered to be about 'this dumpy little bear that wanders around asking silly questions, making up songs and going through all kinds of adventures, without ever accumulating any amount of intellectual knowledge or losing his simple-minded sort of happiness' (Hoff, 1982, p. xiv). At another level, it is a very appealing narrative about trying to make sense of a world that is full of surprises, and full of understandable wisdom – an example, as Hoff demonstrates, of 'Western' Taoism.

Some treasures of literature have a moral that is not only explained and deliberately exploited, but also, in its awesome circumstances, brings the narrative home to us, with a lingering afterthought. Such stories are forgotten only with difficulty, if ever. The story of 'two foolish children in a flat who most unwisely sacrificed for each other the greatest treasures of their house' (Henry, 1960) is probably one such literary gem. In Henry's short story, *The Gift of the Magi*, the wife cuts off her long beautiful hair, with the intention of selling it to obtain money to buy her husband a chain for his ancestral watch. He, on the other hand, sells his watch, given to him by his father, in order to buy his wife a comb for her long hair! The story is not new, it has a familiar ring, and we groan with anticipatory recognition of the plot, but few of us, having read the story, with its lilting colonial americanisms, will ever look at a fine comb for long hair in the same way again. The story becomes part of the narrative of *our* lives. Not only do we recognize the plot, but we continue to remember the wonderful use of the English language. Thus, 'Had the Queen of Sheba lived in the flat across the airshaft, Della would have let her hair hang out the window some day to dry just to depreciate Her Majesty's jewels and gifts' (Henry, 1960, p. 73). The image of this young woman with wonderful long hair, deliberately 'showing off', even to the Queen of Sheba, not only tickles our fancy, but vicariously, in so many other ways, we realize that we have been there, done the same thing, or certainly wished we had! The narrative tells us much about human nature in a gentle and whimsical fashion. Imagine now as a nurse having to shave Della's hair, for brain surgery. Imagine now Della's hair falling out due to chemotherapy. It is the power of the narrative in literature not only to highlight a specific story, but also to enable us to change and think differently, due to the force of the narrative, even in other unconnected instances.

Similarly, Jim, Della's husband, displays the same amusing human quality of wanting to show off that which we pride. Thus, 'had King Solomon been the janitor, with all his treasures piled up in the basement, Jim would have pulled out his watch every time he passed, just to see him pluck at his beard from envy' (Henry, 1960, p. 73). This so human quality is narrated with enormous benevolence, and probably in no small way contributes to our sympathetic approach to the misguided pair – but then, 'life' can be like that.

Not all couples, however, are so overtly in love with each other. Married life is portrayed in literature in all its various forms, from the fatally enamoured youngsters, Romeo and Juliet, so memorably brought to our consciousness by Shakespeare, through to the awful horrors of trapped lives, as portrayed by *Madame Bovary* in the novel of that title by Gustave Flaubert, or *Anna Karenina* in Leo Tolstoy's epic novel, to the consequences of destroyed childhood and youth, as depicted by *Tess of the D'Urbervilles* in Thomas Hardy's tragic English novel. There is no paucity of sad tales concerning marriages, as Tolstoy observed: 'Happy families are all alike; every unhappy family is unhappy in its own way' (Tolstoy, 1875/77). It is one of the properties of literature, that it can help us understand and process the world around us, take the obvious and even ordinary, and help us to see ourselves in a new light.

Anton Chekhov's short story *Grief*, a truly poignant narrative about the life of 'Grigory Petrov, a turner, who had long enjoyed a reputation as an excellent craftsman and at the same time as the most drunken ne'er-do-well in the whole Galchine district' (Chekhov, 1885, p. 15), illustrates superbly the complexity of married life and how it can be misunderstood by others. Not only do outsiders not fully understand the relationship between the drunken husband and abused wife, but the very life of Grigory seems to count for little as indicated by the health care workers he encounters. His narrative to outsiders seems to be insignificant, and yet he himself must have impinged on the lives of the health care workers he met.

Let us therefore look more closely at this story, by way of example, to see what it has to narrate. As the story of one human being, it can be appreciated and understood by all human beings. The narrative is written from the perspective of Grigory, but is not told directly by him. It could well have been written by the nurses on the ward, as a record of his admission to hospital and, therefore, so-called 'nursing history'. Thus 'Grigory remembered that his grief had started the night before' (Chekhov, 1885, p. 17), an observation that hints at some level of temporal insight, but leaves us wondering about the exactness and precision of timing. Grief for Grigory has an acute onset. He later adds that this grief started in fact from the time his wife, 'looked at her bully of a husband as she had never looked before' (Chekhov, 1885, p. 17).

With painful insight, Grigory realized, as we so often do, that something was amiss, but he also realized it too late. He decided to take his ill wife to hospital, despite an impending snow storm. As the storm broke, the snow fell and the horses (which had been borrowed from a neighbour, for the purpose of taking his wife to hospital) refused to walk any further. As he turned around to look at his wife, he realized that she was already dead. Here Chekhov the writer, latter-day physician and natural psychologist notes that 'the turner wept. He was not so much sorry as vexed. His grief had only begun, and now it was all over' (Chekhov, 1885, p. 18). How often, by the time we realize that we must act and start working towards that goal, are we stopped in our tracks by that which we most fear. Grigory was just starting to realize that he really had to begin treating his wife differently, and to grieve for the perfect marriage which had never existed, when his wife died. Now his newly found grief is compounded by fate – for he grieves not only for a failed marriage, or for a meaningful relationship but, realizing it is already all over, he is vexed and cannot put the situation right. Chekhov, with that genius for double meanings and subtle linguistic nuances characteristic of his genre, has Grigory comment to himself, 'What with drinking, fighting, and poverty he had not noticed how life had passed' (Chekhov, 1885, p. 18). Life had indeed passed away for Grigory in terms of missed opportunities in a stormy marriage, but also, intent as he was on driving the horse through the snow towards the hospital, he had not noticed when his wife – his life? – had passed away.

It is only now, realizing that all is over, and in a state of shock, that Grigory begins to query the irrationality of his present actions 'Where am I going?' Grigory asks himself with a start, 'I have to make arrangements for her funeral, and I keep driving towards the hospital. I must be going mad.' (Chekhov, 1885, p. 18). This confusion of purpose and intent, so common to those in a state of grieving shock, is a new feeling for Grigory, and he is understandably afraid of his newly discovered loss of control. Loss of control due to alcohol abuse was a familiar feeling to him, but this was something new. He was totally sober, wanted the very best for his wife, and yet fate had dealt him such an awful hand. The numbness of grief and shock really slowed him down. After a lifetime of maltreating his wife and being a rather obnoxious neighbour (we can surmise), he is now alone. He is all alone on the sledge-cart taking his wife to the hospital, and therefore there is no one with him to give moral support or practical advice.

Thus 'He knew he ought to get out of the sledge, but his whole body felt so numb that he could not have stirred even if he were to freeze to death. And so he fell asleep peacefully' (Chekhov, 1885, p. 19). Just as we can conclude the script for Henry's short story about Jim and Della, so we can imagine what lurks behind this awesome Russian phrase 'to freeze to death'. It is one of the well-known hazards of heavy drinking in Central Europe, and especially in Russia, that every winter, after a heavy night's frost, there is a gruesome catch of corpses to be taken to the county morgue. In drunken stupors, alcoholics lie down, to sleep themselves peacefully to a frozen death. In this instance, the irony is that Grigory is not drunk – so many times he had been, but not this time. Now he is intoxicated with grief, numb with despair and disbelief. Sleep is a blessing – and tomorrow, as always, is another day.

Grigory wakes up in the local hospital. He is in shock and pain, and realizes that something is not altogether right. 'What's the matter with my legs, Sir? My arm?' 'You can say goodbye to your arms and legs. You got them frozen. There, there. . . . What are you crying for? You've had your life, haven't you? You must be sixty if a day – isn't that enough for you?' (Chekhov, 1885, p. 20). This conversation, so typical that we have all heard it before, suddenly hits us with an enormous force. We have listened to Grigory's narrative, identified with him, seen the world through his eyes – and therefore this conversation seems to us to be not only paternalistic and insulting, but also missing an important point. Grigory has gangrenous arms and legs, which need to be amputated. As a turner he needs healthy limbs, and only as a turner can he start to pay back his neighbour money for the horse (which of course has died in the snowstorm). His wife is dead, he is in debt, and he is now also disabled. However far-fetched the story may seem to a modern urban reader, it is neither that original nor that specific to one people or one culture. In addition, today, pulled from the brink of death, many a would-be Grigory might not even be conscious but rescued only to survive in the hazy world of persistent vegetative state. The devastation and horror of the situation would be imposed on the family, rather than the patient. Just as Grigory was not sure whether he would have been better off left for dead, frozen in the snow, so many a relative wonders whether it would have been better to have let their family member die.

This short story, named *Grief* by Chekhov, is a masterpiece of psychological insight and a narrative so rich that its implications linger on long after the closing of the last page. The use of such stories to illustrate psychological truths and to help nurses appreciate 'stories of our lives' is obvious. Inasmuch as this particular narrative has the qualities of an epic legend, where it is beyond time and culture and we can both identify with it and accept it as our own story (or at least the story of someone who is part of the narrative of our own life), we can echo, mindful of Grigory's fate, Warner's comment on homecoming, that, 'We're all wayfarers and make our own destinations as we go' (Warner, 1994, p. 94).

Nursing and life's narrative

As with other professional disciplines, the pre-registration education of nurses is so prescribed that nursing students have little opportunity to examine literature and the humanities and how these may impinge on nursing. The current call for nurses to start reading literature and utilizing the rich wisdom contained in the humanities is therefore predominantly a call to qualified nurses. Although it is often nursing lecturers who advocate that nurses should read more literature, in order to see how they can benefit professionally from examining the literature, it is qualified nursing practitioners who appear to be in the best position to appreciate the imperative and to appreciate the benefit of the humanities for nurse education.

Currently, however, nurse educators are calling for just such an increase in the coverage of humanities in the pre-registration nursing curriculum; they have in mind a greater integration of the humanities into basic nursing education. Such integration, despite the limitations placed on pre-registration curriculum design, seems to be a good way forward in that the humanities can be nicely woven into the fabric of nursing theory, and superbly reflect aspects of nursing practice. Some nurse educators talk about the 'tapestry of care' (Gendron, 1994), and indeed weaving 'narratives' and the humanities into aspects of nursing theory and practice seems to be not only achievable but also aesthetically pleasing and psychologically well grounded.

Nurse educators consider the humanities and specifically the use of literature to be useful educational approaches that widen horizons and illuminate the realities of living (Watson, 1993/94; Darbyshire, 1994a,b; Brykczyńska, 1995). The aspect of nursing which so many nurses find hidden in the study of humanities is interpersonal caring. It is the aspect of caring contained in literature which intrigues nurses and is the subject of an increasing volume of literature. Nurses look at several types of caring contained in several forms of literature and the arts. There is great European and World literature, which is read for its portrayal of universal values and for the treasures of psychological insight which are contained within it, such as the short stories of Chekhov. There is also, increasingly, literature written by nurses and social scientists about nursing and patients, which is definitely full of the caring 'gems' that the nurse educationalists are looking for (Hudson Jones, 1988; Styles and Moccia, 1993; Watson, 1993/94; Jones, 1995).

Nurses, when they read literature and take to studying the humanities, consider the studied arts from at least two perspectives. On the one hand there is the sheer enjoyment of the studied art, a celebration of felicity that something can be so beautiful, moving or poetically phrased. On the other hand, there is an appreciation of the content of the art, which illustrates a way of caring. Needless to say, these two approaches can and often do overlap, and whereas the first approach is open to ever wider interpretations and therefore more potentially engaging, the second approach can actually be limiting if, in the search for the so-called 'caring gems', the context and aesthetic quality of the narrative are overlooked or considered to be of secondary importance.

To look at art and the humanities with the sole aim of examining what they can tell us about 'caring' is rather constraining. The arts, if they are truly 'great', will always in some way reflect what matters in our life, and what matters in our life will always to some extent demonstrate what we care about, what we care for, and how and why we organize our living the way we do. Caring is inherently portrayed in great art, because we have at the very least evidence of the caring executed by the artists, who demonstrate in their art a concern not only for technical perfection and artistic truth but also a wish to share these insights in a tangible way. Furthermore, in order for something to be considered great art, it needs to demonstrate an interest in something meaningful to the narrative of our life – some aspect of caring. As Hugo Meynell comments, in his monograph on aesthetics, 'A great novel or play should deal with important rather than trivial matters seems to confirm to commonsense notions of what it is for a work of literature to be great' (Meynell, 1986, p. 50).

This idea that art 'naturally' demonstrates caring is not without its critics. However, Meynell continues in his passage on the lack of triviality in art, 'A great poem could hardly be concerned with what is not of central importance in human life, or be morally indifferent or frivolous in attitude' (Meynell, 1986, p. 75). While this is undoubtedly part of the argument, there is also much evidence that it is precisely in attention to small details and the idiosyncrasies of life, many of which are amusing and superficially trivial, that an artist can transform an ordinary passage of prose into a great piece of literature, or transfigure a painting like any other into something memorable and unique. Perhaps what is so special about great art is that, without being pretentious, it *can* portray the ordinariness of our lives, warts and all, full of the natural, inherent humour of life, and make it wonderful.

There are many paintings of Christ preaching to the crowds, a religious subject which in itself is very ordinary. In a small etching by Rembrandt held in the National Collection of the Smithsonian Institute in Washington DC, this familiar scene is represented for us once again. What makes this etching so memorable, however, is not only the technical excellence of its execution, but primarily the attention to detail. This detail is frivolous and certainly secondary to the primary subject matter and yet, precisely because it is not essential to the subject matter, it transforms the etching from a rough sketch to a great piece of art. Christ is standing on some steps, around him a crowd is gathered, listening attentively, and in the foreground a young child is playing with its toy. How often we see children, supposedly in a world of their own and not 'paying attention' at all to the adults surrounding them, and yet how often we later find out that they retained everything that was going on. Like old ladies quietly knitting as they listen to someone telling a tale, so children who are apparently absorbed in their own pursuits can retain all that is said and all that is going on around them. This etching demonstrates the attention Rembrandt payed to the smallest details of ordinary life – it is its authenticity that hits home so hard and makes it memorable and elevates this otherwise plain line drawing from a mere representation to a thing of beauty and a work of art. Here attention to the 'trivial' and possibly frivolous by Rembrandt is exactly what makes this etching so memorable. It is the 'little things' that matter.

The notion that the truth of our lives can be reflected in the arts has been examined in depth. Inasmuch as it is precisely the reality of our lives that is seen as a worthy subject for art, it can be said to be beautiful. Surely this particular human way of being must be true for us, and the more in touch we are with our humanness the more honest we become with ourselves, and upon examining this humanness of ours, we find it to be true and also beautiful. Rembrandt's etching was beautiful, also because it was 'true'. Children are like this and crop up everywhere, even where we would not expect them. The etching had a truth to convey and was also therefore found to be beautiful.

The connection between truth and beauty is superbly brought out in a recent, highly readable book on art and theology by the Bishop of Oxford, Richard Harries (1993). However, it is the New England poet, Emily Dickinson, who so succinctly captures the interrelationship, recounting that:

'I died for beauty, but was scarce
Adjusted in the tomb,
When one who died for truth was lain
In the adjoining room.'

(Dickinson, 1960, p. 54)

The newly dead soul enquires of his 'soul-mate' what brought them there, only to find out that they died for truth. Emily Dickinson concludes that 'the two are one; we brethren are.' Thus if indeed there is an aspect of truth that is inherently concerned with beauty, because truth is beautiful, then what makes up the essence of truth is also caught in the net. Thus not only are lofty subjects worthy of great art, portraying what we care about, but so also are the everyday, ordinary and mundane. That is also part of us, part of the truthful story of our lives, and therefore also beautiful.

There is one possible exception to this, namely, how does one define as beautiful (because it is 'truthful') those aspects of our lives which are simultaneously hurtful, painful or broken, not to mention violent or evil. Even if the artist can beautifully capture these areas of our 'ordinariness', how does one accommodate, for example, the truthful, realistic art of Lucien Freud, or the alarming frank brutality of Freda Kahlo? Even well-intentioned art, such as that of Susan MacFarlane exhibited in England during 1995, portraying aspects of cancer care for women with breast cancer, can appear uncaring and questionably 'beautiful' to some people, although it apparently portrays a particular type of accepted and 'lived' reality. For some women, care for breast cancer must be transposed from the plane of the awful and hideous to at least the plane of the acceptable and personal. Whether this truth about themselves can ever be seen as beautiful is something only they can say in their own narratives. And it is their narrative above all else which will be beautiful, being their story – certainly not their disease or their pain.

None the less, when an artist, poet or writer can capture these brutal truths and make them beautiful, they become memorable and can start to reshape our professional insights. It is poets rather than professionals who mostly manage to capture the hurts and brutalities of life, and paradoxically make them beautiful and therefore acceptable aspects of our being. Emily Dickinson notes, concerning the nature of pain, what nurses have been saying for years, but she says it poetically, with a lived experience of personal knowledge and reflection:

> Pain has an element of blank;
> It cannot recollect
> When it began or if there were
> A day when it was not. . .

This is an extremely accurate description of psychic pain, and possibly of chronic pain of long duration. The onset of this pain is lost in the depth of perception's timelessness. Dickinson adds:

> It has no future but itself,
> Its infinite realms contain
> Its past, enlightened to perceive
> New periods of pain.

> (Dickinson, 1960, p. 75)

There is here a feeling of hopelessness and despair tinged with an aspect of considered knowledge. Pain is like that – without beginning or end, enlightening in itself! How often we ask the patient to 'describe' the pain, where description is based on experience and only feeds future expectations. More than a description of transient, expected pain, as would be the case after elective surgery, this is a description of an endless pain, possibly without obvious cause, and certainly unwelcome.

Finally, it is a function of art to state the obvious, but in such a way that we feel we have either never considered reality in that way before, or never seen beauty in the ordinariness of our lives quite like that before. T. S. Eliot, in his poem *Little Gidding* (1979, originally published in 1944) within the *Four Quartets* states, as many nurse educators intuitively feel, that all too often:

> The end of all our exploring
> Will be to arrive where we started
> And know the place for the first time.

We have now seen how literature can demonstrate and play before us the entire range of human emotions and human tales. The end point that we have reached is an understanding that we are all vulnerable and never really know what is around the corner. As we proceed through the narratives of our own lives, we affect the narratives of others, and attempt to create final destinations, in mutual dialogue. As the wise nurse Virginia Henderson observed, 'good nursing calls for a willingness on the nurse's part to selectively express what she is feeling and thinking so that a mutual understanding may develop between nurse and patient' (Henderson, 1991,

p. 34). Literature promotes the expression of feelings and thinking and can help the mutual understanding which leads to 'nursing's' caring dialogue.

This approach is rarely used in the sciences, but is commonly encountered in the arts and humanities. We explore ideas contained in the humanities, not only to come up with totally new insights, which would be a nice bonus, but to go through a reconfirming process, through familiar territory, to emerge where we started from and realize that we have changed. The story is the same, the painting stays unaffected by the comments of the viewer – but we change, and start looking at the world differently.

Conclusions

All of nursing takes place in the context of a story, the story of at least two lives, the life of the nurse who is nursing and that of the patient who is being 'nursed'. The humanities have for centuries concerned themselves with recounting, retelling and re-examining the many-faceted aspects of human living and human stories. The purpose of scrutinizing our lives in this way is to give them meaning, to be able to articulate sense and significance where this would otherwise be impossible for the ordinary person. As Shakespeare so eloquently commented, in one of his sonnets, poetically expressing ourselves can 'give sorrow words that grief can never speak'. Meanwhile, at the other end of the scale, joy and exuberance are often the domain of the musician or sculptor.

It is one of the qualities of the arts that they *can* mirror our feelings, reflect the nature of our lives and, characteristic of all truly great, beautiful art, change us for ever. It is a characteristic of art that it can change the story of our life. It is within the domain of the humanities that the arts which reflect our realities and often try to reshape them, and the philosophical arts which try to bestow meaning on our lives, most appropriately reside. If the humanities are such a treasure trove of resources concerning human nature and humanness, why is it that nursing, which so studiously pursues physical, psychological, sociological, anthropological and even moral theories, appears to neglect the 'arts' and 'philosophy' – the very foundation of all the other disciplines and sciences? Are not art and literature nursing's distant mirror?

References

Barthes R (1977) *Image Music Text*. Fontana, London.
Bettelheim B (1976) *The Uses of Enchantment: The Meaning and Importance of Fairy Tales*. Penguin, London.
Brykczyńska G (1995) Humanism: a weak link in nursing theory? In Schober J and Hinchliff S (eds) *Towards Advanced Nursing Practice: Key Concepts for Care*, pp. 111–32. Edward Arnold, London.

Chekhov A (1885) Grief. In *Lady with Lapdog and Other Stories*, pp. 15–20. Penguin Classics, Harmondsworth.

Cooper A and Harpin V (1991) *This is Our Child: How Parents Experience the Medical World*. Oxford University Press, Oxford.

Danto A (1981) *The Transfiguration of the Commonplace*. Harvard University Press, Cambridge, MA.

Darbyshire P (1994a) Understanding caring through arts and humanities: a medical/nursing approach to promoting alternative experiences of thinking and learning. *Journal of Advanced Nursing* 19, 856–63.

Darbyshire P (1994b) Understanding caring through photography. In Diekelmann NL and Rather ML (eds) *Transforming RN Education: Dialogue and Debate*, pp 275–90. National League for Nursing, New York.

Dickinson E (1960) *Selected Poems*. The Laurel Poetry Series, Dell Publishing Co., New York.

Downie RS (ed.) (1994) *The Healing Arts: An Oxford Illustrated Anthology*. Oxford University Press, Oxford.

Eliot TS (1979, originally published in 1944) *Little Gidding – The Four Quartets*. Faber and Faber Ltd, London.

Gendron D (1994) The tapestry of care. *Advances in Nursing Science* 17, 25–30.

Harries R (1993) *Art and the Beauty of God*. Mowbray Press, London.

Henderson V (1991) *The Nature of Nursing: Reflection After 25 Years*. National League for Nursing, New York.

Henry O (1960) *Short Stories*. Everyman's Library, JM Dent and Sons Ltd, London.

Hoff B (1982) *The Tao of Pooh*. Methuen Press, London.

Hudson Jones A (ed.) (1988) *Images of Nurses: Perspectives from History, Art and Literature*. University of Pennsylvania Press, Philadelphia.

Jones L (1995) *Handle with Care: A Year in the Life of Twelve Nurses*. Macmillan Publishers, London.

Jury M and Jury D (1976) *GRAMP*. Grossman/Viking Press, New York.

Kansuke N (1976) *The Silver Spoon* (translated from Japanese by Etsuko Terasaki). Chicago Review Press, Chicago.

Leininger M and Watson J (eds) (1990), *The Caring Imperative in Education*. National League for Nursing, New York.

Meynell H (1986) *The Nature of Aesthetic Value*. Macmillan Press, London.

Moyle W, Barnard A and Turner C (1995) The humanities and nursing: using popular literature as a means of understanding human experience. *Journal of Advanced Nursing* 21, 960–4.

Patrick J (1995) Giving the Knowledge. *Nursing Standard* 9, 20–1.

Radsma J (1994) Caring and nursing: a dilemma. *Journal of Advanced Nursing* 20, 444–9.

Ree J (1987) *Philosophical Tales: An Essay on Philosophy and Literature*. Methuen and Co., London.

Sheppard A (1987) *Aesthetics: An Introduction to the Philosophy of Art*. Oxford University Press, Oxford.

Styles M and Moccia P (eds) (1993) *On Nursing: A Literary Celebration – An Anthology*. National League for Nursing, New York.

Taylor B (1994) *Being Human: An Ordinariness in Nursing*. Churchill Livingstone, Melbourne.

Tolstoy L (1875/77) *Anna Karenina* (translated by Edmonds R, 1969). Penguin Books, Harmondsworth.

Warner M (1994) *Managing Monsters: Six Myths of Our Time: The Reith Lectures 1994.* Vintage Press, London.
Watson J (1988) *Nursing: Human Science and Human Care – A Theory of Nursing.* National League for Nursing, New York.
Watson J (ed.) (1993/94) *Aesthetics and Nursing Theory.* National League for Nursing, New York.
Wilde O (1993, originally published in 1888) The devoted friend. In *The Happy Prince and Other Stories*, pp. 67–92. Wordsworth Classics, Ware.
Zalumas J (1995) *Caring in Crisis: an Oral History of Critical Care Nursing.* University of Pennsylvania Press, Philadelphia.

Further reading

Begley A-M (1995) Literature, ethics and the communication of insight. *Nursing Ethics* 2, 287–94.
Downie RS (ed.) (1994) *The Healing Arts: an Oxford Illustrated Anthology.* Oxford University Press, Oxford.
Styles M and Moccia P (1993) *On Nursing: A Literary Celebration – An Anthology.* National League for Nursing, New York.

5

Competency-based continuing education: a model to promote caring in critical care

Carol Cox

In the vast professional literature on caring, relatively little space is devoted to looking at the skills that are needed in order to be able to care 'safely'. The skills most likely to be mentioned are empathy and communication – both extremely important, but all the empathy and communicative skills in the world will not be sufficient for a nurse to minister to a patient caringly in an intensive-care unit. This chapter therefore looks at the types of skills and competencies that might be needed, how they might be promoted, and how their acquisition might be evaluated and monitored. Nursing care is about competencies to practise – within the framework of all ethical imperatives to care, and an increased sensitivity to the distress of patients. It is a basic tenet of nursing that, in order for holistic care to be provided, the nurse must first be appropriately skilled and proficient at what he or she is doing. This is the starting point and the motivation for a search for a more sensitive caring approach. Nowhere is this issue so important or does it reflect the wisdom of nursing so much as in the highly technologically controlled environments of intensive-care units, where compassion will be evident through a striving to ensure appropriate intervention.

Introduction

The purpose of this chapter is to discuss the promotion of caring through the development and implementation of a competency-based continuing education model in critical care. The chapter will articulate how the development and implementation of a competency-based continuing education model can support nurses in their quest to provide competent quality care. A review and critique of the literature is included, as the historical background highlights the theoretical perspective for developing a competency-based continuing education model that promotes caring. The rationale and method for the model, which are based on del Bueno's (1978) competency-based continuing education process, are derived from research (Cox, 1993) conducted in an attempt to promote caring by improving nursing competence in a critical-care environment. Caring is associated with competent practice and is considered to be the core of nursing (Leininger, 1984; Ritchie, 1992; Radsma, 1994). Furthermore, in society caring is regarded as a form of protection, responsibility and a charge to health-care professionals (Webster, 1989; Greenleaf, 1991).

The need for nurses to develop and maintain competence is important, as the nursing profession is increasingly involved in litigation (Kinney *et al.*, 1988; Duffield, 1991). In an effort to promote quality care, nurses are required by health-care institutions to provide evidence of completion of formal course work in continuing education in order to practise in specialty areas (Shuldham, 1986). Emphasis on ongoing educational development is essential in view of the fact that human resources are a valuable commodity in the provision of quality nursing care (Alspach, 1982, 1984; del Bueno and Altano, 1984; Scott, 1984; Kinney *et al.*, 1988; Duffield, 1991). Nurses represent the highest proportion of health-care employees within the critical-care environment, and are a resource that should be highly regarded and valued. To assist nurses in their desire to provide quality nursing care, educational programmes must be developed that ensure an appropriate and adequate level of competence within an ever-changing technological environment.

The English National Board for Nursing, Midwifery and Health Visiting has established specific criteria for specialist courses in critical care (English National Board for Nursing, Midwifery and Health Visiting 1990a,b) with the intention of developing practitioners who will demonstrate effective competence and provide high-quality nursing care. However, not all nurses who work in critical care have access to these courses. Therefore, another form of educational model must be made available to these nurses in order to facilitate the development of competence that will lead to the provision of high-quality care.

The continuing education model discussed in this chapter addresses a means for achieving competence in any area of practice identified by nurses. Inherent within the model is the ability to integrate clinical and didactic components of the curriculum and simultaneously to create a collaborative information-sharing environment. Assessment of competence is criterion-referenced and evaluated procedurally through direct observation. The most viable approach to the measurement of competence at this time is the observation method, combined with a performance checklist (Bower *et al.*, 1988; Waltz *et al.*, 1991). Assessment of competence should be objective in nature.

Objectivity in the assessment of competence and testing is essential

(Alspach, 1984; Bower *et al.*, 1988; Curzon, 1990; Walklin, 1991; Waltz *et al.*, 1991). Curzon (1990) indicates that an objective test is one in which every question is set in such a way as to have only one correct response, and that the term 'objective' relates to the assessment process. Walklin (1991) further indicates that objectivity is reflective of quality, validity and reliability within any system of assessment and accreditation. An accreditation process confirms the existence of particular competencies and gives credit for them. The methods agreed by the assessor and the one being assessed are critical if subsequent awards are to be credible. However, the abilities to be tested involve examiners, who are human beings, and therefore decisions may to some extent be subjective in their nature, unless extreme care is taken when assessment strategies are developed.

Seedhouse (1986, 1991) indicates that high levels of objectivity are often assumed to be impossible, and that 'values permeate everything'. Seedhouse further indicates:

> The view that any inquiry, even 'scientific inquiry', can be detached, impartial, and objective is incorrect. In all inquiry the unquantifiable, human, creative, emotional, intuitive, caring, egoistic, competitive element is indispensable. . . . The idea of 'total objectivity' (in any given situation) is a myth which can be shown to be so once and for all, with a consequent emphasis on our shared humanity.
>
> (Seedhouse, 1991, p. 95)

Discussions associated with objectivity (Brown, 1985; Davis, 1985; Seedhouse, 1986, 1991; Munhall, 1989; Waltz *et al.*, 1991; Yin, 1994) reflect the fact that standards must be met in an attempt to achieve an objective perspective. Traditional views of objectivity involve a detached attitude, which draws on the best features of genuine inquiry. Objective inquiry is considered to be impartial. Impartiality is difficult to achieve; therefore another sense must be added if an evaluation is to be realistic. This sense is the consensus view, or the 'subjective' perspective as reflected by the participants who are involved in the assessment process and their interpretation of the participant's performance. Within this chapter inter-rater reliability will be considered as a method for moving closer to objectivity in assessment.

A perspective regarding reliability, validity and interpretation has been postulated by Walklin (1991). Performance-based assessment in the work environment involves candidates demonstrating competence under varied conditions. Assessment and confirmation of competence, either simulated (laboratory) or actual (whilst care is being given), means the collection and evaluation of evidence about the performance of an individual by an observer. For such assessment to be 'objective', reliable and valid, the observer must consistently and accurately exercise his or her judgement. Reliability and validity of observation can be facilitated by standardizing assessments against agreed objectives and criteria. Accreditation of competence confirms the existence of knowledge and skills and gives credit for proficiency. Bazinet *et al.* (1989) agree with Walklin that assessment methods and criteria should be agreed upon by the assessor and the candidate for an award of competence to be credible.

One arena for competency development and observation of competence is the critical-care environment, which is fraught with crisis, emergencies, high patient acuity and an unrelieved atmosphere of urgency and tension that may, by the very nature of the setting, colour the perspective of the observer. Davis (1985) has analysed the process of observation in natural settings, which entails how to observe objectively, when to observe, and what to observe in relation to field research. The observation method in the assessment of competence has many similarities to those of field research. Davis identifies the process of conducting field research as 'participant observation research' (Davis, 1985, p. 48). Within the discussion, the role of the known observer is highlighted. Here, the participant observer is always more or less active, that is, asking questions, carrying on informal and formal conversations, and interacting at strategic moments with those being studied. The very act of being involved, rather than just watching and listening in the presence of human situations, influences the interpretive perspective of the observer. For a sense of 'objectivity' to be achieved, there must be an agreed view amongst all, or almost all, of the participants within the study (Seedhouse, 1986, 1991).

Review of the literature

This literature review will consider the historical background related to competency development. Competency-based orientation programmes will be reviewed and critiqued. National Vocational Qualification perspectives will be discussed in relation to del Bueno's (1978) criteria, and the English National Board's requirements for developing expertise in clinical practice will be addressed. These discussions underpin the theoretical perspective and rationale for use of a competency-based continuing education model to promote caring within the work environment of critical care.

Background

A review of the literature shows that many approaches can be used to design a competency-based continuing education model for nurses. Since the late 1970s and the work of del Bueno (1978) on competency-based education, the emphasis has shifted from traditional education programmes to competency-based education programmes in health-care institutions, industry, colleges and universities in the USA (Van Druff, 1974; Spady, 1977; del Bueno, 1978; Boyer, 1981; del Bueno *et al.*, 1981; Ghiglieri *et al.*, 1983; Porter, 1984; Selfridge, 1984; Flewellyn and Gosnell, 1985; Hagerty, 1986;

Schamaus, 1987; Ferraro, 1989). Prior to the writings of del Bueno (1978), competency-based approaches were associated with teacher (Houston and Howsam, 1972; Hyland, 1990), dietitian and pharmacist (Hart, 1976) education. Competency-based orientation programmes in nursing have been co-ordinated by hospital staff development departments since the early 1980s in the USA (del Bueno and Kelly, 1980; Boyer, 1981; del Bueno *et al.*, 1981; del Bueno and Altano, 1984; Haggard, 1984; Ferraro, 1989; Benedum *et al.*, 1990). Specifically in critical-care nursing, the benefits of competency-based orientation programmes have been discussed (Alspach, 1982, 1984; Freeman *et al.*, 1983; Porter, 1984; Scrima, 1987). However, active implementation of competency-based programmes is still in the early stages of development in nursing (Snyder-Halpern and Buczkowski, 1990).

Many types of environment may be classified as critical care. Intensive care, cardiovascular surgery, accident and emergency, high dependency, theatre, post-anaesthesia recovery units, burn, trauma and cardiac departments, to name but a few. The literature review conducted did not specifically reveal the use of a competency-based continuing education model in critical care, either as it relates to orientation or to continuing education in the UK.

Snyder-Halpern and Buczkowski (1990) and DiMauro and Mack (1989) postulate that at this time in nursing history, nurses are feeling confused and disorientated within the acute-care environment as technology changes rapidly. The complexity of role development in nursing requires an orientation/precepted phase (United Kingdom Central Council for Nursing, Midwifery and Health Visiting, 1994) and continuing education programme to develop and update competencies that will lead to quality outcomes in patient care.

Within the current hospital climate in London, there is an increasing pressure to contain costs whilst maintaining quality patient care (Harrison, 1992; Tomlinson, 1992). Creative measures must be employed which will effect cost-effective care and staff-nurse retention, and that will promote caring. Traditionally, nursing staff development/continuing education programmes have been targeted towards meeting basic external agency requirements for fire and safety, cardiac and pulmonary resuscitation and specific general learning needs of new employees. Specific programmes targeted towards competency development and assessment have not been the rule in acute-care settings (Bazinet *et al.*, 1989; Snyder-Halpern and Buczkowski, 1990; Angelucci and Todaro, 1991). Furthermore, according to Angelucci and Todaro (1991) and Snyder-Halpern and Buczkowski (1990), the effectiveness of centralized programmes in enhancing clinical competence is uncertain and debatable because the above-mentioned educational experiences are typically conducted as general classroom activities and are usually provided during institutional orientation only. Education to performance relationships are difficult to measure under these circumstances, as the allowance for individual nurse learning needs in association with competency development cannot be addressed within a generic centralized approach. Therefore, a decentralized competency-based continuing education model is required to provide information about relevant topics, and to assess performance during skill acquisition (Snyder-Halpern and Buczkowski, 1990; Angelucci and Todaro, 1991; Polis, 1992).

In competency-based education, the stress is on performance and not merely knowledge gained. The following five characteristics of competency-based education, identified by del Bueno (1978), should form the foundation of a competency-based education model:

- the focus is on outcomes;
- statements are criterion-referenced;
- the acquisition of learning is flexible;
- a fixed sequence of learning is absent;
- the relative values of each outcome are considered.

Schamaus (1987) indicates that competency-based education is well suited to nursing because nursing is practice-based. The emphasis within the educational programme is on adult-learning principles and the incorporation of performance criteria. The focus of Schamaus' work is orientation within the theatre environment. Within the theatre, each nurse entering orientation brings a variety of experiences and skills. According to Schamaus it is essential that each nurse participates in defining his or her own learning needs.

Criterion-referenced performance outcomes in competency-based education provide each nurse with an explicit, value-based list of expected behaviours and process elements to comprehend better his or her learning needs in the context of the working environment (Ferraro, 1989). According to Ferraro, the criterion-referenced structure guides the assessor's evaluation of the observed behaviours in the appropriate clinical setting. Each nursing ward/unit identifies its own performance standards to be assessed on the basis of its patient population, standards of care, policies and procedures, and the daily activity and demands of the ward/unit. In addition, in order to provide flexibility in learning and skill acquisition, a variety of learning tools must be at the nurse's disposal.

Competency-based orientation programmes

DiMauro and Mack (1989) have designed a competency-based orientation programme for the clinical nurse specialist. The purpose of the programme is to facilitate role transition, as newly appointed clinical specialists have unclear ideas about how to establish themselves in their new role, regardless of whether they are experienced or inexperienced. Role conflict arises when the clinical nurse specialist's preconceived role expectations do not conform to the reality of the way in which the role must be performed.

Factors that have been identified as affecting role development include previous work experience, educational background, personal expectations, and the orientation process. Competencies in each of the four above-mentioned role components have been specified. These components were based upon the observation of actual performance of experienced clinical nurse specialists. The competencies are related to specific outcomes. For example, within the education role component, the competency-outcome statement is: 'incorporates adult learning principles into meeting educational needs of staff' (DiMauro and Mack, 1989, p. 76). Broad competency statements are subdivided into areas of criteria, evaluation and resources. The evaluation structure for the competency of incorporating adult learning principles into meeting educational needs of staff is 'verbalization of knowledge to clinical nurse specialist/preceptor' and a 'self-assessment questionnaire' (DiMauro and Mack, 1989, p. 76). A needs-assessment tool is also completed by the staff nurse, and presented to the clinical nurse specialist or preceptor.

If del Bueno's (1978) criteria for competency-based continuing education are used as a reference point for DiMauro and Mack's (1989) model, a measurement system for how educational needs have been met would need to be incorporated into the programme. A review of the competency-based orientation programme for clinical nurse specialists could give rise to concern regarding reliability and validity. The literature associated with DiMauro and Mack's orientation programme fails to substantiate how the programme has been validated, or how the criteria which underpin the four role components were established. There has been no discussion regarding the reliability of the programme, or how and whether reliability has been determined. Reliability and validity, and how they have been determined, are important components of a competency-based continuing education programme. Analysis reveals that the programme is subjective in its assessment method and does not meet the specific criteria outlined by del Bueno (1978) as procedurally based, and also relative values are lacking for an objective assessment to be conducted.

Peterson (1991a,b) has developed a competency-based orientation programme for a cardiovascular surgery unit at Georgetown University Hospital, Washington, DC. Competencies are focused on outcomes, criterion-referenced and process-orientated. A partial example of a competency, determined for admission of a cardiac surgery patient to the unit, which is process-orientated is as follows: (1) set up monitor, transducer, and tubing for standard pressure lines; (2) set up cardiac output tubing; (3) set up suctioning devices, orogastric, endotracheal, chest suction; (4) set up ECG (Peterson, 1991b, p. 17).

Although Peterson's (1991a,b) competency-based orientation programme is far more exhaustive than DiMauro and Mack's (1989) model in terms of process elements, it does not meet all of the criteria delineated by del Bueno (1978). Statements are not criterion-referenced in all instances, and relative values for each outcome have not been considered. Some competencies begin to reflect a procedure orientation for assessment purposes; however, the structure is not consistent. Therefore, objectivity cannot be achieved in assessment. In addition, concerns regarding the reliability and validity of Peterson's (1991a,b) competency-based orientation programme may also be raised. It has not been clearly identified how the programme has been validated in relation to development of the competencies.

Bazinet *et al.* (1989) have also developed a competency-based orientation programme for critical care. The rationale for developing the programme was based on the length of a centralized orientation programme, cost and consumption of resources. Use of multiple orientation assistants for one orientee created difficulty in maintaining communication and contributed to an inordinate duration of progress through orientation. Each orientation assistant wanted to assess skills which had been previously assessed by another orientation assistant. In addition, no mechanisms were established to individualize orientation for the orientee. Regardless of the level of experience of the orientee, each was treated equally as they progressed through a regimental programme. The rigidity of the programme, with its emphasis on structured classes to provide all content, frustrated the experienced critical-care nurse.

A 'priority matrix' as suggested by del Bueno (see del Bueno 1982, cited in Bazinet *et al.*, 1989, p. 69) was used to give priority to identified skills requiring proficiency development. Within the matrix, the importance of each competency and the frequency of use in the clinical area were identified. Competency was defined as the 'possession of required knowledge, skills and abilities' (Bazinet *et al.*, 1989, p. 70). The programme developed for orientation has become a special designation for an educational approach centred on clear expectations defined in behavioural terms, accountability and individuality. The emphasis is on performance, and is procedurally orientated for evaluation purposes.

Bazinet *et al.* (1989) chose to consult JoAnn (Grif) Alspach, RN, MSN, in the development of their competency-based orientation programme. The structure suggested by Alspach follows her 1982 and 1984 process for developing a competency-based orientation programme (Alspach, 1982, 1984). The process specifies the following.

1. Competencies should:
   (a) delineate one set of integrated/complex behaviours (e.g. for assessment);
   (b) be clearly written;
   (c) reflect the framework of nursing care delivery (e.g. nursing process);
   (d) reflect RN role description.
2. Performance criteria should:
   (a) be an essential or mandatory aspect of performance (e.g. standards of practice);
   (b) be converted from solely cognitive to include measurable clinical behaviours.

3. Learning options should include actual experience in performing the behaviour stated in the criteria.
4. Evaluation mechanisms:
    (a) tools should be designed to reflect the performance criteria directly;
    (b) written tests should be constructed to evaluate cognitive performance criteria.
5. In developing the list of competencies and performance criteria, the writers should:
    (a) avoid using educational jargon;
    (b) streamline and simplify the format to include each competency statement and its accompanying performance criteria (e.g. procedure orientated);
    (c) delete terminology reminiscent of objectives;
    (d) validate competencies and performance criteria with each unit head nurse (ward sister) and staff (especially orientation assistants – preceptors).

(Bazinet *et al.*, 1989, p. 71).

Bazinet *et al.* (1989) postulate that they have used del Bueno's (1978) criteria to design their competency-based orientation programme. Analysis reveals that the programme meets all of the criteria except those within the domains of outcome and evaluation. The specific competencies do not appear to be outcome-orientated or value-referenced. Furthermore, if the programme is critiqued in terms of qualitative research methodology, its accuracy and credibility may be questioned. Within the literature, Bazinet *et al.* (1989) have failed to identify how each criterion has been determined. From a quantitative research perspective, the reliability and validity may be questioned. No reference has been made to the methods utilized to achieve reliability and validity of the programme, or even whether the criteria were considered.

Although Alspach's (1982, 1984) structure is credible in terms of process, the structure does not include del Bueno's (1978) outcome orientation, unless outcome is assumed to be inherent within the nursing process. Unfortunately, the above-mentioned element is not clarified within the literature associated with either Alspach (1982, 1984) or Bazinet *et al.* (1989).

National Vocational Qualifications

Following the publication of the 1986 White Paper, the National Council for Vocational Qualifications was established with a remit to design and implement a national framework for vocational qualifications. The securing of national vocational competence can be discerned from the early activity of the Training Agency (Hyland, 1990), which featured prominently in the New Training Initiative of 1981. The origin of the approach, according to Hyland (1990), can be traced to research and development in Performance-Based Teacher Education in the USA in the 1960s.

National Vocational Qualifications (NVQs) are qualifications that establish the standards for occupational and professional competence. According to the National Council for Vocational Qualifications (NCVQ) (National Council for Vocational Qualifications, 1992a,b,c), NVQs are practical, relevant to today's market and valued by employers. Established awarding agencies such as City and Guilds are changing their qualifications so that they can meet the new NVQ criteria and become NVQ centres. New NVQs are also being developed in occupations for which no qualifications had previously existed.

NVQs are composed of units which specify in detail the standards to be achieved and the performance criteria associated with the standard. An area of work and a level of proficiency locates it within the NVQ framework. The overall framework reflects how qualifications relate to each other and how individuals may progress through the NVQ system. The National Council for Vocational Qualifications publications indicate that NVQs have removed previous barriers to learning and the achievement of qualifications. One advantage is that NVQs have no 'unnecessary entry requirements, no prescribed method of delivery, no time limits for achievement, and no age limits' (National Council for Vocational Qualifications, 1992a, p. 3). Furthermore, a feature of the NVQ system is flexibility with a range of learning and assessment services such as individually tailored programmes, open learning and modular packages. Assessment consists of assembling a range of evidence of achievement. Standards for the NVQs are stated in the units of competence, and therefore the learners and trainers know what standards are expected within the assessment.

A review of the NVQ competencies and assessment strategies for healthcare assistants for the North East Thames Region (Care Sector Consortium, 1992) indicates that colleges offering the NVQ programmes meet most of the fundamental criteria recommended by del Bueno (1978). Elements of competence have been specified which are criterion-referenced, outcome-orientated, and value-based. Self-reflection as discussed by Schon (1991) is a key element within the assessment strategy. In addition, knowledge is assessed by written examination and discussion, and performance is assessed by the evidence of direct observation by a trained assessor, and documentation provided by the learner (e.g. completed observation charts, and intake and output records).

Flexibility has been identified as a major advantage of the NVQ programme (National Council for Vocational Qualifications, 1992a). However, an examination of learning schemes within colleges offering NVQ programmes shows that learning is specified and assessed within specific time frames (Cox, 1993). Although individuals participate in goal setting, assessment is regimented, and all performance criteria must be assessed according to a predetermined schedule.

Ward (1990a,b,c) has commented on the NVQ system. The National Council for Vocational Qualifications has established core skills under three headings (Groups One to Three) which underpin competent performance in most activities, regardless of occupation. Core skills within Group One are problem-solving, communication and personal autonomy (which includes recognition of one's own strengths and weaknesses, a responsibility for self-development, working in a team or group, and self-evaluation) (Ward, 1990b). Group Two core skills, which are not universally required according to Ward (1990b), cover the application of mathematics, foreign language and information technology competence. Group Three core skills include economic and industrial understanding, environmental education, education for citizenship, health education, scientific and technological understanding, career education and guidance, and aesthetic and creative knowledge. Core skills should be expressed in outcome terms, and should be capable of recognition in a wide variety of educational and vocational programmes. Statements of core skills should also be defined in a way that separates them and identifies them as being independent of other statements of competence. However, Ward (1990b,c) has identified difficulties in delivery of the NVQ programme. A great deal of thought will be required as to the purposes of identifying core skills and the way in which they are delivered and recorded. Ward (1990a,b) indicates that it would be contrary to the whole spirit of NVQs to mandate success in a core skills unit if the skills do not have a direct relevance to competence within the occupation specifying NVQ.

Furthermore, Ward (1990b,c) expresses concern regarding the understanding and knowledge which are important elements within competency development. Many of the contributors to papers addressing knowledge begin with the assumption that what matters most in competence development programmes is that knowledge and understanding are important only in the contribution that they make to underlying principles and not to practical application (Ward, 1990b). Contributors are not agreed as to what constitutes understanding and knowledge, or whether it matters that there should be a generally agreed definition. A consensus view is that, within vocational qualifications, the focus should not be on the recall of facts, but on the understanding and application of knowledge in practical situations. Within the NVQ system, flexibility allows for a purist view in which assessment of competence is separated into observation on the job, and assessment of knowledge by examination. Assessment mechanisms within the purist perspective have not incorporated the assessment of knowledge and understanding within practical performance. Therefore, Ward (1990b) envisages that, in some programmes, there is a gap between what can be practicably observed in the workplace and the means of knowledge assessment.

Ward's (1990a,b,c) commentary raises theoretical questions which need to be addressed within the NVQ system as it relates to practical examples. Although there has been mention of a need for validity and reliability in assessment, and that traditional measures of performance are not appropriate for a standards-based programme, little has been done to establish measures which are appropriate and determine the reliability and validity of NVQ programmes (Unwin, 1990; Ward, 1990b).

A reiteration of the National Council for Vocational Qualifications (1992a) position on barriers to access and mode of education and training underpins Unwin's (1990) article on staff development and competence through NVQ. Unwin addresses the college environment in particular, and indicates that the NVQ is a statement of competence that 'describes a person's ability to perform to specific standards under normal working conditions, and that a specified time to be spent in education, training or work must occur before the award can be made' (Unwin, 1990, p. 26). Concern is expressed by Unwin regarding the colleges' ability to deliver NVQs successfully. According to Unwin, research suggests that for colleges to deliver NVQs successfully, substantial changes must be made in three areas. The areas identified through the research are the approach to curriculum design and pedagogy; the clientele colleges provide for; and the management style and organization. Changes should not be developed in isolation, but should evolve within inter-college working groups which explore the implications of NVQs for all members of staff within the college. New roles and competencies for staff members are required, as well as a commitment from all levels within the college setting. That commitment must begin with the Principal.

One of the significant changes within the college setting is that departments and individuals can no longer 'plough their own furrow' (Unwin, 1990, p. 28). All members must function as part of a team providing an integrated learning environment so that students may work towards competence within a range of occupationally based modules. Many of the module elements may be common to more than one department within the college. The nature and design of NVQ programmes has a major impact on teaching staff, and their responsibility for delivering the programmes.

Unwin (1990) and Merritt (1990) suggest that the self-contained classroom in which the teacher delivers a subject-based course via the traditional approach must disappear. The focus must shift from input methods of teaching to outcomes, that is, competencies demonstrated under working pressures. Individual action plans must become the teaching mode in order to enable colleges to deliver NVQ programmes effectively. Therefore, teaching staff must rethink the curriculum and the methods by which learning and assessment opportunities are presented.

Merritt (1990) also proposes that the quality of learning programmes depends not only upon the learning materials selected for use, but also on the extent to which access, support and guidance are provided. The assessment and learning schemes which underpin the NVQ must take place in a suitable environment which can maximize choices for students, enhance their learning experiences, and develop the desired outcomes in terms of competence.

English National Board's requirements

The English National Board for Nursing, Midwifery and Health Visiting has established criteria for specialist courses in critical care (English National Board for Nursing, Midwifery and Health Visiting, 1990a,b) as well as many other specialist areas. The purpose of specifying the curriculum content is to ensure the efficient and appropriate education of nurses. The curriculum content allows the educational programme to be based on the nurse's individual learning needs, and is structured so as to provide nurses with the knowledge and skills required for them to function competently within a minimal amount of time. Polis (1992) has suggested that this type of educational structure is ideal for competency development.

The English National Board *Cardio-Thoracic Nursing* (1990a) and General *Intensive Care Nursing* (1990b) reflect identical aims, which are to enable registered nurses to become competent to assess, plan, deliver and evaluate the specialized nursing care of patients undergoing treatment within the specialty area being studied, and to give support to relatives and staff. Entry requirements for both courses are identical, as is course length (24 weeks, 900 hours in length, exclusive of annual leave; in addition, not less than 40 days, 300 hours, shall be allocated to the theoretical component). The guidelines for curriculum development for each course are identical within the common core. Common core themes have been outlined so that multiple nursing specialties can be brought together for learning purposes. The Board intends that the common core themes shall form a part of the course foundation and continue to do so to course completion (English National Board for Nursing, Midwifery and Health Visiting, 1990a,b). The course design should be flexible enough to allow for the provision of shared teaching and learning opportunities. Core themes include

> social, political, cultural and environmental issues, legal and ethical issues and responsibilities, concepts of health, health promotion and education, exploration of the health–illness continuum, nursing theories and models of care, applied anatomy and physiology, applied microbiology, pathological processes, diagnostic, therapeutic and technological developments, resources, quality assurance, information management, educational role and responsibilities, applied research studies, and personal development.
> (ENB, 1990a, p. 3; ENB, 1990b, p. 3)

Learning outcomes specify that upon completion of course ENB 249 the nurse will be able to do the following:

1. demonstrate the ability to utilize theories of nursing in order to select an appropriate strategy for the management of nursing care;
2. apply an in-depth knowledge and understanding of the relevant applied anatomy, physiology and pathology of the cardio-pulmonary systems to nursing care;
3. demonstrate the ability to identify the complications that may arise

following trauma, surgery and/or changes to the cardio-pulmonary function, and take appropriate action;

4. facilitate rehabilitation by effective health promotion, enabling a return to independence and adoption of a healthy lifestyle;
5. demonstrate understanding of the ethical and moral issues surrounding resuscitation (English National Board for Nursing, Midwifery and Health Visiting [ENB], 1990a, p. 4).

Upon completion of course ENB 100 the nurse will be able to do the following:

1. utilize theories of nursing in order to select an appropriate strategy for the management of nursing care;
2. apply in-depth knowledge and understanding of the normal physiological processes and subsequent changes as a result of critical illness;
3. demonstrate understanding of the complex issues involved in the care of the critically ill and be able to assist patients, relatives and/or friends to make informed choices where this is possible;
4. perform effectively in the acute/emergency situation and adapt to the changing needs of the patients;
5. enable patients to progress from varying degrees of dependence towards independence or to a peaceful death;
6. demonstrate an understanding of the special needs of children in an adult intensive-care environment, based on the concept of family-centred care;
7. perform effectively in the multi-disciplinary team (ENB, 1990b, p. 4).

Although there are variations in wording, the two courses are similar in learning outcomes, covering a broad context within the specialty area. Competency/proficiency in assessment, planning, implementation and evaluation of nursing care is evident in all outcomes; particular emphasis is evident in ENB 249 (ENB, 1990a, pp. 2 and 3) and in ENB 100 (ENB, 1990b, pp. 2–4).

Practical experience (8 weeks, 300 hours) is specified for both courses within a training institution which offers the specialty in nursing. Subsequent practical experience is also identified as 'supervised practice' within the course members' own Health District (ENB, 1990a, p. 4; ENB, 1990b, p. 4; ENB 1990c).

A review of curriculum documents for two colleges of nursing associated with the ENB 100 course and ENB 249 course reflect similar learning outcomes to those of the English National Board (Cox, 1992). However, a stronger emphasis on pathophysiology and development of clinical competency is evident in the ENB 100 course. Examples of the learning outcomes for the ENB 100 course are as follows:

- develop and reinforce the knowledge and skills necessary to provide skilled nursing management of the patient receiving respiratory support;
- differentiate between the physiological mechanisms of normal neurological functioning and the effect of pathological disturbances caused by trauma;
- participate in measures taken in intensive care to control the spread of infection;
- identify the predisposing factors which may cause acute renal failure and utilize techniques which will render a biochemical/fluid balance, based on individual patient needs;
- utilize alternative methods for inducing relaxation and reducing pain in critically ill patients (Cox, 1992).

Examples of the learning outcomes for the ENB 249 course are as follows:

- demonstrate an understanding of the particular health-care needs of various client groups with cardio-thoracic conditions;
- demonstrate an understanding of environmental issues which may contribute to the development of respiratory or cardiac disorders and their implications for health care;
- demonstrate an understanding of the provisions and effectiveness of screening measures and health education in cardio-thoracic care;
- demonstrate an understanding of how clients' lives may be affected by having a cardiac infection (Cox, 1992).

Interviews conducted over a period of 3 months amongst staff nurses, ward sisters, clinical tutors and course directors who had completed and/or were teaching the ENB 100 and 249 courses indicated that there were mixed opinions about the ability of the ENB courses to provide adequate opportunities for the participants to achieve the competency level each envisaged would be reached as a result of taking the course (Cox, 1992). An additional form of educational model was considered to be essential in order to develop and maintain competence within the critical-care environment.

Competency-based continuing education model

The competency-based continuing education method which follows is underpinned by del Bueno's (1978) criteria. The advantages and disadvantages associated with the method are reviewed, and data collection methods and the reasons underlying the choice of data gathering tools are explained. In addition, credibility, accuracy, validity and reliability are addressed in relation to inter-rater reliability.

Educational methodology

In order to obtain a clearer understanding of the competency-based approach to continuing education, two educational methodologies will be reviewed – pedagogy and andragogy.

Pedagogy is an educational methodology which is most familiar to educationalists (Knowles, 1978, 1980, 1984). For centuries this method has been the exclusive approach to education. The pedagogical method evolved from early European monasteries where monks taught young children simple skills. Originally, the primary skills taught using the pedagogical approach were reading and writing. Pedagogy was adopted and reinforced by missionaries in the eighteenth and nineteenth centuries as elementary schools spread throughout much of the world. By the turn of the century, when educational psychologists began to study learning scientifically, a stronger contribution to the pedagogical approach was made. This was achieved primarily by limiting research to child reactions to didactic teaching. Until the advent of adult-learning theory (Knowles, 1980), shortly after World War Two, there was a paucity of knowledge about reactions to learning.

Following World War Two, educators recognized that the basic approach of pedagogy, which was the transmission of knowledge and skills, was insufficient for adult learners. Adults wanted more than fact-laden lectures, rote memorizing and examinations. New knowledge was being conceptualized and discovered, technological changes abounded, and mobility of the population became a way of life. In addition, there were massive economic and political changes. Knowledge gained at one point in time became obsolete within a matter of a few years. Therefore it became impossible to define education solely as a knowledge transmission process, and it became redefined as a lifelong endeavour of continuing enquiry. Consequently, according to Knowles (1980), it is most important to develop the skill of self-directed learning.

Andragogy shifts the focus away from didactic lectures towards self-directed learning. A series of structured activities is planned that enables the learner to acquire knowledge and skills appropriate to the learning desired. It is a practical approach which is job-related and that emphasizes the value of the training programme to work performance (Knowles, 1984). Within adult-learning theory, the suggestion is made that the maturation process amplifies the differences between individuals (Knowles, 1978; Tornyay and Thompson, 1987). It proposes that adult learners prefer instructional situations that allow them to be self-directing, actively involved, able to use past experiences in new learning situations, and able to manage current life situations and problems effectively.

The twentieth century has been an era of knowledge explosion, technological revolution and economic opportunity. Therefore the contemporary approach to education must be to produce a competent individual. The most effective approach to producing a competent individual is to promote the acquisition of knowledge and skills in the context of application. This new mode has particular relevance in the field of adult education (Tornyay and Thompson, 1987). Adults must learn to live productively in a world in which change is accelerating (Knowles, 1984). The andragogical method facilitates this process.

The competency-based approach

A competency-based approach to continuing education is consistent with the andragogical model. It is a non-traditional, outcome-orientated educational method that is responsive to adult development needs and learner readiness. An underlying assumption within andragogical theory is that, given the opportunity to study and absorb the continuing education materials, followed by practical experiences, adults will learn without a structured classroom situation (del Bueno and Altano, 1984). Self-paced learning is important within the andragogical approach. Self-pacing incorporated into learning recognizes that students learn at different rates, and encourages and allows them to use the amount of time needed to reach the stated competency outcome. According to Tornyay and Thompson (1987), self-pacing is closely aligned with mastery of competencies, and closely associated with placing the responsibility for learning on the learner.

The learner who is using a competency-based approach to continuing education must be motivated, self-directed and actively involved in the continuing education process. Emphasis is placed on what the learner can do and what he or she knows on completion of competency-based continuing education. This is in contrast to the traditional education model. del Bueno and Altano (1984) suggest that traditional education emphasizes what a learner should know at the end of a continuing education programme.

Competency – a definition

Competency is operationally defined as the integration of the knowledge, skills and attitudes required for performance in a designated role or setting in relation to predetermined criteria (Skelton, 1989). The learner in a competency-based continuing education programme is educated to demonstrate the knowledge and proficiencies critical to a given skill, function or profession. For the nurse within the critical-care environment, competence in clinical situations which involve patients is the desired outcome (Alspach, 1984).

The role of the educator

The educator within a competency-based continuing education programme is a facilitator of learning, and not a provider of content (del Bueno, 1978).

The nurse in the critical-care environment is directed to the proper resources and materials by the educator. Content acquisition is accomplished by the nurse learner independently. The educator assists the nurse learner in achieving specific outcomes or competencies through actual application and skill attainment. Time previously spent on lecturing in the traditional model is used to individualize clinical learning experiences and identify performance problems. The primary concern of the educator is to assist the nurse learner in meeting the criteria necessary to achieve proficiency in competency performance.

The environment for learning

The environment for learning within a competency-based continuing education programme is the actual clinical area. The emphasis shifts from 'know that – knowing about' in the classroom to 'know how – knowledge application' in the real world (del Bueno *et al.*, 1981; Alspach, 1984). According to del Bueno and Altano (1984), the concentration of learning within the clinical environment reduces the time it takes for the nurse to become competent and to feel comfortable with his or her acquired proficiency and knowledge. Time is used more efficiently in the clinical setting, where learning is applied and subsequently reinforced as a result of increased exposure to patient care.

Purpose and process

Emphasis on competency performance defines more clearly the components of nurse development and their relationship to variables within the context of patient-care delivery. Implementation of a competency-based programme, and in particular del Bueno's (1978) process, will have a major influence on changing nursing care (del Bueno *et al.*, 1981; Lassiter-Kroslak *et al.*, 1985; Flatley-Lunde and Durbin-Lafferty, 1986; Snyder-Halpern and Buczkowski, 1990). Nurses demonstrate their expertise at a defined level of practice, role and setting. Proficiencies required within the field of critical-care nursing are distinguished from those required in another field through the process of planning, implementing and evaluating the competency-based continuing education programme. Alspach (1984) postulates that it is not enough merely to verbalize a description of a given situation – the nurse must demonstrate knowledge and proficiency.

Successful completion of the programme, or components of it, is documented by an assessor as the nurse learner demonstrates competent performance behaviours in the essential aspects of the critical-care nursing role. As a result of collaboration, the staff nurse, educator, assessor and ward sister share common goals and expectations in the educational process.

Model development

Development of a competency-based continuing education model begins with an examination of the philosophy of the nursing management team and nursing staff. The patient population and clinical experiences should be reviewed in order to identify essential competencies inherent within practice. The sequence of steps to follow (Figure 5.1) for derivation of competencies is initiated in a situational analysis, which is an analysis of all external and internal factors that impact or will impact on the clinical area. Subsequent to the situational analysis, general learning statements of proficiency and performance criteria can be synthesized. Learning tasks contained within these general statements are matched to the criteria forming competency statements of aims (assessment), objectives (implementation) and evaluation. Standards for process and outcome are written in tandem with the competency statements. A matrix (del Bueno, 1989) indicating the priority for skills requiring proficiency development should be delineated.

An inventory of competencies (Figure 5.2) which are normally performed within the critical-care environment, their criteria and process elements underpinning the competencies and standards of practice should be derived from reviews of the literature associated with the clinical environment (e.g. intensive care or accident and emergency nursing). Once the competencies have been identified with their underlying assessment criteria and process elements, these are written in the form of competency assessment sheets and standards. Each competency and its standard should be written separately, so that each can be assessed individually.

In order to substantiate the credibility of the competencies and standards, each competency and standard should be analysed by expert nurses from at least two similar nursing care environments. Following development of the competency assessment forms, accuracy of rating can be substantiated through test–retest within the critical-care environment using additional expert nurses as assessors and assessees in role–role reversal. This process substantiates inter-rater reliability in relation to objectivity and accuracy in assessment.

Credibility and accuracy are as essential as validity and reliability. Credibility is subject orientated in association with truth value, and underpinned with the criteria of member checking, peer examination and structural coherence (Krefting, 1991). Accuracy is associated with representation, in that it reflects how closely the competencies fit actual practice. However, a difficulty in the critical-care environment is that there are few controlling variables. Accuracy can be determined in the naturalistic setting by assessing how well the competencies, as delineated in process criteria, are performed under varying conditions.

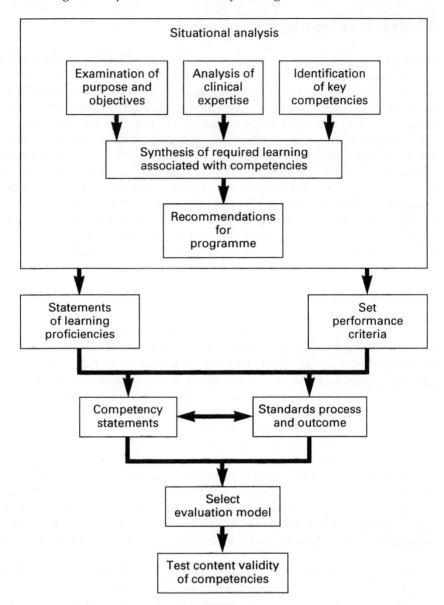

Figure 5.1   Development of competencies process.

Nurse identification of learning needs and goals

Competency-based continuing education (Figure 5.3) is directed towards the end achievement rather than the means of instruction. Therefore the approach to learning is flexible in methodology. Competencies, as identified

The Critical-Care Competencies Inventory is designed to determine knowledge and proficiency needs related to your nursing practice in Critical Care/Coronary Care. Each item on the the inventory is followed by a choice of possible responses: 0, 1, 2 or 3. Please read each item carefully and decide which choice best rates your level of knowledge/proficiency. Indicate your rating by ticking the box corresponding to your choice. Please respond to every statement. If you are not completely sure which response is most accurate, put the response which you feel is most appropriate for your needs. It is important that you rate each item as honestly as possible. All information obtained from the inventory will be treated with the strictest confidence.

0 = no theory or experience
1 = theory – but little or no experience
2 = limited experience – needs assistance
3 = have experience and feel comfortable with level of competence/performing

Years or months of experience as a Critical Care Nurse: _____

Please identify all ENB courses you have completed:

Competency	0	1	2	3
Cardiovascular system:				
Arterial line				
set up				
Arterial blood sampling –				
Drawing blood from an A-line				
Apical pulse auscultation				
S-1				
S-2				
S-3				
S-4				
Murmurs				
Blood pressure				
Doppler				
Palpation				
Peripheral pulses				
Dorsalis pedis				
Posterior tibial				
Popliteal				
Femoral				
Radial				
Brachial				
Carotid				
Central venous pressure				
Set up CVP				
Read CVP				
12-lead ECG				
Can set up and perform 12-lead recording procedure				
Can interpret normal 12-lead				
Can interpret abnormal 12-lead				
A-line wave-form interpretation				
Swan Ganz				
PA line set up				
Wedging				
Interpreting PAS/PAD/PAM (normal and abnormal)				
Can identify normal and abnormal waves				
IABP-datascope – assist with set up				
Temporary pacemakers –				
preparation for insertion of pacemaker				
Assisting with procedure				
Care of patient with temporary pacemaker				
Care of pacemaker equipment				
Connection of patient to lead wires				
Operate and set rate and output (mA)				
Determine threshold				
Overdrive				
Set up asynchronous (fixed rate) and synchronous (demand)				

Figure 5.2 Critical-Care Competencies Inventory (sample of one page).

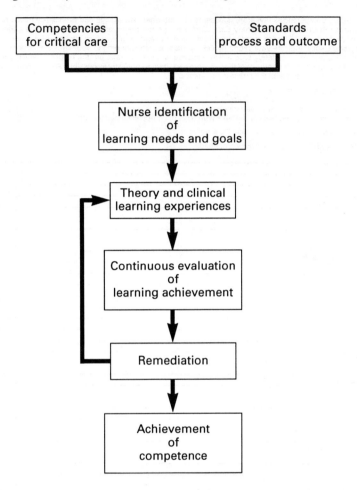

Figure 5.3   Competency-based continuing education model.

by the nurse, are completed on the basis of the sequence, method and pace that best fulfil the individual needs and preferences of the nurse. Simulated (laboratory) situations are arranged prior to actual performance by the educator and nurse. According to Alspach (1984), simulated situations should occur whenever learning experiences might be potentially dangerous to the patient. The nurse may choose to use the laboratory assessment column on the competency assessment sheet to assess himself or herself reflectively, or to request a peer to assess and provide feedback prior to the actual clinical assessment.

Evaluation in competency-based continuing education

Evaluation methods in competency-based continuing education structures are criterion-referenced. The nurse is assessed against a set of criteria specified as standards for a particular competence. By comparing performance with the criteria, the assessor determines the adequacy of the performance by assigning a safe or unsafe tick in the check-list column (Alspach, 1984; Battenfield, 1986; Cox, 1993). Criterion-referenced evaluation formats facilitate performance appraisal for the educator, assessor, ward sister and the nurse. The nurse can identify his or her own progress and areas that require remediation. In addition, the competency assessment forms may be used to document experience and continuing education.

del Bueno and Altano (1984) and Alspach (1984) have indicated that interpersonal and critical thinking skills cannot be measured with criterion check-lists. Therefore only the cognitive and psychomotor domains are assessed by the use of certification competency sheets. Performance evaluation of attitudes and values, according to Knowles (1980), is less precise and more difficult to assess than knowledge and skill. Evaluation of learning within the affective domain is best accomplished in simulation situations that involve critical thinking, role-playing and decision-making (Knowles, 1980). Within the competency-based continuing education programme, simulated laboratory experience may be used to assess attitudes and values.

Identification of learning needs

For the purpose of determining areas for developing or improving competence, a competencies inventory form should be designed. The inventory should incorporate a weighting scale in its format, so that it serves as a good tool for identifying areas for competence development and may also be correlated with previous inventories or with direct observation of performance within the critical-care environment. As indicated previously, competencies for inclusion on the inventory can be gleaned from the literature on critical-care nursing. Following compilation of the competencies which cover all major aspects of care, a panel of expert nurses should be asked to review the list and select the competencies which are most applicable to the nursing care provided within the speciality.

The strength of the competencies selected for the inventory is not based solely upon choice of the design, but is also influenced by the amount of control that exists within the indices of the conceptual variables (competencies) identified on the inventory. When control is applied to measurement, it refers to the ability of the inventory to index the concepts (competencies) with precision, accuracy and sensitivity (Mishel, 1989). The inventory is a questionnaire. Precision refers to the preciseness or exactness with which the inventory defines the competency. Accuracy refers to the correctness, sometimes referred to as truthfulness, with which the inventory (questionnaire) defines the competencies, and sensitivity refers to the ability of the inventory to discriminate between different levels of competencies. Mishel (1989) suggests that a precise, accurate and sensitive questionnaire will provide more control within a study, leading to a clearer interpretation of the findings. The determination of competencies for inclusion on the inventory is a form of study undertaken in order to develop a precise, accurate and sensitive tool for use in determining areas of competence that require development or refinement. Therefore, to achieve the above-mentioned objective, the percentage of agreement (Giovannetti and Mayer, 1984; Bower *et al.*, 1988) can be calculated for each competency selected by the panel members for inclusion on the final instrument.

Inter-rater reliability can be substantiated by a percentage of agreement method. Inter-rater reliability refers to the consistency of ratings among different levels of competencies. Individual judgements come into focus in selecting competencies for inclusion on an inventory (questionnaire). These judgements are subjective and are known as 'value judgements', and they depend entirely upon the perspective of the individual who is selecting the competencies for inclusion on the questionnaire. When a number of individuals are selecting competencies, inter-rater reliability measurements are important. The percentage of agreement measures the level of reliability between raters related to each competency. Generally, agreement of 90 per cent or more is considered to be standard for a competency to be included on a questionnaire. However, an agreement of 80 per cent is considered by many researchers to be acceptable (Giovannetti and Mayer, 1984).

Rating scales provide a sound method by which to evaluate clinical proficiency both qualitatively and quantitatively (Bower *et al.*, 1988). Rating scales work well with a norm-referenced approach to assessment and evaluation, and numerical values can be assigned to each rating category. The following categories are recommended for delineation on a competencies inventory:

0 = no theory or experience;
1 = theory – but little or no experience;
2 = limited experience – needs assistance;
3 = have experience and feel comfortable with the level of competence/ performing.

Following development of the competencies inventory, each member of the expert nurse panel should answer the inventory in order to validate content and construct. Content validity refers to the sampling of the content area (competency) being measured, and is based on the individual judgements of raters. To determine content validity, a systematic examination by a panel of experts will ensure that the competencies listed adequately represent required nursing competencies. Construct validity concerns the appropriateness and adequacy of the variables (competencies) within the inventory, and how they are quantified.

Following validation of the inventory, it should be piloted on a group of nurses within the nursing care environment. The purpose of the pilot is to substantiate the credibility and validity of the inventory. Each nurse in the pilot group should be asked to complete a brief questionnaire indicating the time and amount of difficulty he or she experienced in completing the inventory. The purpose of the questionnaire associated with the inventory is to identify any further areas requiring refinement that may have been missed by the expert nurse panel.

Development of the competency-based assessment tools and standards associated with care provided in the critical-care environment should follow the same process for validation as the inventory. A pilot of each tool should be carried out before the tools are finally used in the competency-based continuing education programme. For ease of assessment, a standard of measurement should be identified. Measurement standards can be identified for laboratory (practice) as well as actual clinical performance. Accepted criteria, as standards of measurement, are safe and unsafe practice (Cox, 1993). Nurses can determine during the assessment process whether the competency being performed and the knowledge/rationale for practice articulated is safe or unsafe.

Implementation of the competency-based continuing education programme

In the first phase of implementation, nurses who will be used as assessors should be orientated to their roles as assessors through a series of discussion and assessment practice sessions. The purpose of orientating the nurses to the role of assessor is to establish their identity and ability as content specialists. A content specialist assesses performance behaviours associated with the criteria validated as items of measure on the competency assessment sheets. Through orientation to the rating process, nurses merge their critical judgement and interpersonal relationship skills. Critical judgement and interpersonal relationship skills are important elements in the assessment of competence (Alspach, 1984), and the reliability of assessed competence is dependent upon critical judgement skills. Each assessor should be knowledgeable about the rating process and procedural skills and knowledge required for a competency to be performed safely. Interpersonal relationship skills form the foundation of *esprit de corps* in interactions between individuals and groups. A positive interpersonal relationship may instil confidence in a nurse who is being assessed. Assessment of competence may be viewed as threatening to some nurses – a nurse who feels threatened, although competent, may be unable to perform successfully in an assessment situation. Positive feedback, reassurance and the appearance of a relaxed attentive assessor can do much to allay apprehension.

Inter-rater reliability is important in assessment of the competence of staff nurses. Raters/assessors are provided with the conceptual definition of the variables to be measured on the competency assessment sheets through the standards (of practice) which support each competency. Content specialists (assessors) should independently rate each other's performance, using the competency assessment sheets, prior to actual assessment of the nursing staff's competence.

Inter-rater reliability is determined by two assessors who rate another nurse's performance simultaneously. Their assessments are then compared for agreement. The assessments continue in role–role reversal until all of the content specialists have had an opportunity to determine their level of rater reliability. A target of 80 to 90 per cent inter-rater reliability should be determined by nursing staff prior to rater assessment. Proficiency and objectivity in assessing competence can be established through the inter-rater process. Criterion-referencing facilitates the opportunity for reflection and objectivity in assessment of performance, because of its domain status. The domain status consists of the procedural elements of the predetermined criteria associated with the performance standards. When criterion-referencing is used in measurement, the emphasis is transferred to what a nurse can or cannot do, or what he or she knows or does not know, and not on how the nurse compares with other nurses.

Staff nurses should be orientated to the competency-based continuing education and assessment process. All staff nurses independently determine their learning and developmental needs by rating their perceived level of competence on the inventory. These ratings serve as a guide for selecting initial competency areas for learning and development. Nurses should be encouraged to participate in the (performance) competency assessment process, so that they can evaluate their own level of competence prior to being assessed by an assessor. Self-selection of competencies and the opportunity to be self-directed in the learning process are important factors in a competency-based continuing education approach (del Bueno, 1978; Cox, 1993).

During actual practice and acquisition of competence, staff nurses may use their peers and/or ward sisters/charge nurses to analyse their performance. This is best undertaken by the peer and/or ward sister/charge nurse observing their practice and rating them in the laboratory column of the competency assessment sheet. Through an emphasis on self-paced learning and the use of educational resources such as multi-media, simulated laboratory practice and review of literature, the model becomes multi-dimensional in developing competence.

Operational support is needed to ensure the availability of resources for learning. Instructional supports should be made available to assist nurses in attaining competence. An assurance that it is not mandatory for nurses to be assessed at a specific time, and that they can wait until they feel ready to be assessed will reduce apprehension and promote learning. If nurses do not succeed when they are being assessed, remedial and/or alternative forms of instruction should be made available. Assessment can be attempted repeatedly until competence is achieved.

The competency-based continuing education model is based on the belief that adults need to be responsible for their own learning and its pace. In del Bueno and Altano's (1984) article, it is acknowledged that it is not easy for a traditional educator to assume the unconventional skills required in a competency-based approach to learning and skill acquisition. This may be said of some nurse managers as well. Revising and relinquishing established patterns of teaching and the expectations of nurse managers may cause physiological and psychological stress. For some teachers and nurse managers, the optional methods of learning and flexible sequencing, and the self-paced nature of the programme, may be difficult to internalize. Therefore these teachers and nurse managers may be unable to accept a competency-based approach as a method for promoting caring.

Conclusions

Within this chapter, competency-based continuing education has been reviewed and a model for the development of competence that promotes caring has been articulated. Competency-based continuing education is a method of informing practice and developing and improving knowledge and performance through a theoretical framework of variable learning which links theories of education and learning. Research indicates that there is a need for nurses to develop and maintain competence in clinical practice (Cox, 1993). Competency-based continuing education will assist nurses in their desire to provide quality nursing care, which is a fundamental premise of caring.

The benefits derived from a competency-based continuing education programme will not eliminate all practice issues which arise within the clinical environment. The approach to education and learning is non-traditional, and unfamiliar to some nurses. Nurses who have been educated in the traditional mode may exhibit resistance to change. A passive learning role is familiar, and may therefore be a more comfortable style for some adults. Therefore, a certain amount of resistance should be anticipated and appropriate measures taken to facilitate effective change so that learning may take place.

Inherent within a competency-based continuing education programme is certification of competence through the assessment process. The latter validates a specific level of performance and knowledge. The United Kingdom Central Council of Nursing, Midwifery and Health Visiting (1990) has recommended that competence and acquisition of knowledge be documented in a portfolio. Documented validation of competence and knowledge acquisition has become a strong marketing tool which the nurse may use to further his or her career, and upward mobility becomes an opportunity for nurses who are not English National Board certificate holders. Nurses who participate in a competency-based continuing education programme which is based within the work environment may use their documented competency certificates and knowledge acquisition to apply for acquired prior experiential learning within the English National Board Higher Award Scheme. Higher and further education received by the nurse make him or her a more competent practitioner as well as a more marketable product within the caring environment.

References

Alspach J (1982) *The Educational Process in Critical Care Nursing.* C. V. Mosby, London.

Alspach J (1984) Designing a competency-based orientation for critical care nurses. *Heart and Lung* 13, 655–62.

Angelucci D and Todaro A (1991) Blueprint for proficient practice: an adult medical–surgical nursing orientation program. *Journal of Continuing Education in Nursing* 22, 205–8.

Battenfield B (1986) *Designing Clinical Evaluation Tools: The State of the Art.* National League for Nursing, New York.

Bazinet L, Erickson V and Thomas J (1989) Developing competency-based orientation for six critical care units. *Critical Care Nurse* 9, 69–77.

Benedum E, Kalup M, and Freed D (1990) A competency achievement program for direct care-givers. *Nursing Management* 21, 32–5.

Bower D, Linc L and Denega D (1988) *Evaluation Instruments In Nursing.* National League for Nursing, New York.

Boyer C (1981) Performance-based staff development: the cost-effective alternative. *Nurse Educator,* September/October, 8, pp. 12–15.

Brown S (1985) *Issues In Health and Disease.* Unit 14, Course 202. Open University Press, Open University, Milton Keynes.

Care Sector Consortium (1992) *NVQ Units for Health Care Assistants.* Crown Publishers, London.

Cox C (1992) *Situational Analysis.* Unpublished paper, South Bank University, London.

Cox C (1993) *Development, Implementation and Assessment of a Competency-Based Continuing Education Programme in Critical Care/Coronary Care.* Unpublished dissertation, South Bank University, London.

Curzon L (1990) *Teaching In Further Education: An Outline Of Principles And Practice,* 4th edn. Cassell Educational Limited, London.

Davis M (1985) Observation in natural settings. In Chenitz W and Swanson J (eds) *From Practice To Grounded Theory,* pp. 48–65. Addison-Wesley Publishing Company, Menlo Park.

del Bueno D (1978) Competency-based education. *Nurse Educator* 5, 10–14.

del Bueno D (1989) Priority matrix. A conference paper read before the Competency-Based Education Workshop, University of Southern Maine, Portland, Maine, 13 May 1982. In Bazinet L, Erickson V and Thomas J (1989) Developing Competency-Based Orientation for Six Critical Care Units. *Critical Care Nurse* 9, 69–77.

del Bueno D and Kelly K (1980) How cost-effective is your staff development program? *Journal of Nursing Administration* 4, 31–6.

del Bueno D and Altano R (1984) Competency-based education: no magic feather. *Nursing Management* 15, 48–53.

del Bueno D, Barker F and Christmyer C (1981) Implementing a competency-based orientation program. *Journal of Nursing Administration* 11, 24–9.

DiMauro K and Mack L (1989) A competency-based orientation program for the clinical nurse specialist. *Journal of Continuing Education in Nursing* 20, 74–8.

Duffield C (1991) Maintaining competence for first-line managers: an evaluation of the use of the literature. *Journal of Advanced Nursing* 16, 55–62.

English National Board for Nursing, Midwifery and Health Visiting (1990a) *Cardio-Thoracic Nursing*. Course No. 249. Ratcliff and Roper (Printers) Ltd, Worksop.

English National Board for Nursing, Midwifery and Health Visiting (1990b) *General Intensive Care Nursing*, Course No. 100, Ratcliff and Roper (Printers) Ltd, Worksop.

English National Board for Nursing, Midwifery and Health Visiting (1990c) *Post-Registration Courses*. Circular 89/27 AS. Ratcliff and Roper (Printers) Ltd, Worksop.

Ferraro A (1989) Developing a competency-based orientation program: the challenge of a multidisciplinary pediatric unit. *Journal of Pediatric Nursing* 14, 325–33.

Flatley-Lunde K and Durbin-Lafferty E (1986) Evaluation of clinical competency in nursing. *Nursing Management* 17, 47–50.

Flewellyn B and Gosnell D (1985) Comparison of two approaches to hospital orientation for practice efficacy and preferred learning methods of registered nurses. *Journal of Continuing Education in Nursing* 16, 147–52.

Freeman A, McMaster M and Hamilton L (1983) Staff development program for critical care nurses. *Critical Care Nurse* 3, 86–92.

Ghiglieri S, Woods S and Moyer K (1983) Toward a competency-based safe practice. *Nursing Management* 14, 16–19.

Giovannetti P and Mayer G (1984) Building confidence in patient classification systems. *Nursing Management* 17, 33.

Glaser B and Strauss A (1967) *The Discovery of Grounded Theory*. Aldine, Chicago.

Greenleaf N (1991) Caring and not caring: the question of context. In Chinn P (ed.) *Anthology on Caring*, pp 71–84. National League for Nursing Press, New York.

Haggard A (1984) *Hospital Orientation Handbook for Nurses and Allied Health Professions*. Aspen Publications, Rockville.

Hagerty B (1986) A competency-based orientation program for psychiatric nursing. *Journal of Continuing Education in Nursing* 16, 158–62.

Harrison B (1992) *A Proposal for the Dissolution of the Bart's NHS Trust*. Consultation Document, November. North East Thames Regional Health Authority, London.

Hart M (1976) Competency-based education. *Journal of the American Dietetic Association* 12, 616–20.

Houston W and Howsam R (1972) *Competency-Based Teacher Education: Progress, Problems and Prospects*. Science Research Associates, Chicago.

Hyland T (1990) Education, vocationalism and competence. *FORUM* 33, 18–19.

Kinney M, Packa D and Dunbar S (1988) *AACN's Clinical Reference for Critical-Care Nursing*. McGraw-Hill Book Company, London.

Knowles M (1978) *The Adult Learner: A Neglected Species*, 2nd edn. Gulf Publishing, Houston.

Knowles M (1980) *The Modern Practice of Adult Education: From Pedagogy to Andragogy*. Prentice Hall Regents, NJ.

Knowles M (1984) *Andragogy in Action: Applying Modern Principles of Adult Learning.* Jossey-Bass Publishers, San Francisco.

Krefting L (1991) Rigor in qualitative research: the assessment of trustworthiness. *American Journal of Occupational Therapy* 45, 214–22.

Lassiter-Kroslak C, Kearney-Rohmann M and Fell R (1985) Competency-based orientation – an idea that works! *Nursing Staff Development* 1, 68–73.

Leininger M (1984) Caring: a central focus of nursing and health care services. In *Care: The Essence of Nursing and Health,* pp. 45–59. Slack Incorporated, New Jersey.

Merritt R (1990) Open and flexible learning: a response to NVQ. *Learning Resource Journal* 16, 30–5.

Mishel M (1989) Methodological studies: instrument development. In Brink P and Wood M (eds) *Advanced Design in Nursing Research,* pp 238–84. Sage Publications, London.

Munhall P (1989) Qualitative designs. In Brink P and Wood M (eds) *Advanced Design in Nursing Research,* pp 161–79. Sage Publications, London.

National Council for Vocational Qualifications (1992a) *NVQ, NCVQ.* NCVQ, London.

National Council for Vocational Qualifications (1992b) *National Vocational Qualifications and Colleges.* NCVQ, London.

National Council for Vocational Qualifications (1992c) *NVQs and Careers Guidance.* NCVQ, London.

Peterson K (1991a) Competency-based orientation program for a cardiovascular surgery unit, Part 1. *Critical Care Nurse* 11, 32–44.

Peterson K (1991b) Competency-based orientation program for a cardiovascular surgery unit, Part 2. *Critical Care Nurse* 11, 15–40.

Polis S (1992) Competency-based laser education. *AORN* 55, 567–72.

Porter S (1984) Ensuring competence: toward a competency-based orientation format. *Critical Care Quarterly* 7, 42–52.

Radsma J (1994) Caring and nursing: a dilemma. *Journal of Advanced Nursing* 20, 444–9.

Ritchie J (1992) Caring for practice: the value of nurses. *Concern* 21, 26–7.

Schamaus D (1987) Competency-based education: its implementation in the O.R. *AORN* 45, 474–82.

Schon D (1991) *Educating the Reflective Practitioner.* Jossey-Bass Publishers, Oxford.

Scott B (1984) A competency-based learning model for critical care nursing. *International Journal of Nursing Studies* 21, 9–17.

Scrima D (1987) Assessing staff competency. *Journal of Nursing Administration* 17, 41–5.

Seedhouse D (1991) *Health: The Foundations For Achievement.* John Wiley and Sons, Chichester.

Selfridge J (1984) A competency-based orientation program for the emergency department. *Journal of Emergency Nursing* 10, 146–253.

Shuldham C (1986) The nurse on the Intensive Care Unit. *Intensive Care Nursing* 1, 181–6.

Skelton G (1989) Assessment and profiling of clinical performance. In Bradshaw P (ed.) *Teaching And Assessing In Clinical Nursing Practice,* pp 160–74. Prentice Hall, London.

Snyder-Halpern R and Buczkowski E (1990) Performance-based staff development. A baseline for clinical competence. *Journal of Nursing Staff Development,* January/February, 7–11.

Spady W (1977) Competency-based education: a bandwagon in search of a definition. *Educational Researcher* 6, 9–14.

Tomlinson B (1992) *Report Of The Inquiry Into London's Health Service, Medical Education And Research, October*. HMSO, London.

Tornyay R and Thompson M (1987) *Strategies For Teaching Nursing*, 3rd edn. John Wiley and Sons, Chichester.

United Kingdom Central Council for Nursing, Midwifery and Health Visiting (UKCC) (1990) *The Report of the Post-Registration Education and Practice Project*. UKCC, London.

United Kingdom Central Council for Nursing, Midwifery and Health Visiting (UKCC) (1994) *The Future of Professional Practice – the Council's Standards for Education and Practice Following Registration*. UKCC, London.

Unwin L (1990) Staff development, competence and NVQ. *Journal of Further and Higher Education* 14, 26–37.

Van Druff J (1974) Learning labs in adult education. *Adult Education* 9, 72–3.

Walklin L (1991) *The Assessment of Performance and Competence*. Stanley Thornes Publishers Ltd, Avon.

Waltz C, Strickland O and Lenz E (1991) *Measurement in Nursing Research*, 2nd edn. F. A. Davis Company, Philadelphia.

Ward C (1990a) *ABC and Beyond*. EDUCA, No. 102, April, pp. 4–5. Guildford Educational Services, Guildford.

Ward C (1990b) *Core Skills and Knowledge in NVQs*. EDUCA, No. 104, June, pp. 8–9. Guildford Educational Services, Guildford.

Ward C (1990c) *Quality Matters*. EDUCA, No. 105, September, p. 9. Guildford Educational Services, Guildford.

(1989) *Webster's Encyclopedic Unabridged Dictionary of the English Language*. Gramercy Books, New York.

Yin RK (1994) *Case Study Research Design and Methods*, 2nd edn. Sage Publications Ltd, London.

Further reading

Bedford H, Phillips T, Robinson J and Schostak J (1993) *The Assessment Of Competencies In Nursing And Midwifery Education And Training*. English National Board For Nursing, Midwifery And Health Visiting, London.

Gaut D and Leininger M (1991) *Caring: The Compassionate Healer*. National League for Nursing, New York.

6

Patients' experiences of being cared for

Paul Morrison

Caring for vulnerable patients is not easy. Even when the nurse thinks he or she has been relatively caring in his or her approach, the patients often evaluate the work significantly differently. Not enough material is published about patients' perceptions of nursing care interventions, and nurses do not spend enough time analysing what patients are saying, and reflecting on their insights and observations. This chapter is the result of a UK study looking at patients' perceptions of being cared for. It is rich in detail and provides much material for personal reflection. Are the concerns of patients predominantly about technical skills, or are they mainly calling for an increase in empathy and a more sensitive psychosocial approach to care giving? Perhaps patients see the need for a combination of the two perspectives. Certainly one cannot emphasize one aspect to the detriment of the other. Holistic care is best practised where good role models and a conducive health-care environment conspire together to promote deliberate caring strategies – a combination of wise professional forethought and compassionate priority setting which reflects patients' wishes.

Introduction

Nurses provide professional care for people who are unable to care for themselves. The potential for working in a more 'person-centred' way can only be achieved by *understanding* more about the experiences of patients who have received care in a professional context. In this chapter, patients' experiences of 'being cared for' in hospital are described. The detailed picture of the patients' experiences highlights the need for quality psychological care in the hospital environment. The information gathered from hospitalized patients provides an interesting background for reflecting on nursing work, and may ultimately lead to higher levels of individualized patient care. More details about the study may be found elsewhere (see

Morrison, 1991, 1992). A full account of the ideas described in this short chapter can be found in Morrison (1994).

Interviews with patients

The methodological approach used to study patients' experiences in this study was guided by existential phenomenology which is characterized by the goal of trying to study human experience from the point of view of the person being studied (Taylor and Bogdan, 1984; Stevenson, 1987). This approach has become a very popular one in health-care research because it has the potential to be especially useful in the study of professional helping relationships. Kestenbaum (1982) claimed that the use of phenomenologically based health-care research provides a powerful set of techniques for exploring patient and professional viewpoints. He suggested that these different perspectives could help to reshape professional practice and policies.

In the study reported here a sample of 10 patients from medical and surgical wards were asked to talk about their experiences of 'being cared for'. Patients also provided details about the social setting in which 'care' was experienced. The interviews focused on *what* the nurses did for patients and *how* they did their work. The patients/informants were ordinary people who were willing to talk openly about their experiences. The emphasis in this study was on 'ordinary' people as patients.

Patients

All the patients in the study were in-patients in a large teaching hospital.

1. Florence (55 years old) had spent only three days in hospital, but she had had several earlier experiences as a hospital patient.
2. James (67 years) was a retired headteacher and had spent one full week in hospital undergoing a series of tests.
3. Eileen (61 years) was a recently diagnosed diabetic who had spent a full week in hospital after being brought into hospital as an emergency admission.
4. Tim (48 years) had spent several weeks in hospital and had been transferred to another hospital for specialist treatment. When he was in hospital he discovered he had lung cancer, and at one point he thought that he had secondary growths, too.
5. Hugh (28 years) spent a week in hospital undergoing a series of tests which resulted in surgery.
6. George (62 years) had had several previous admissions to hospital, and on this occasion he was in hospital for seven days.

7. Martha (35 years) stayed in hospital for eight weeks because she needed extensive skin surgery. She travelled down from the north of England because the surgeon in this hospital was the 'top man' for this type of surgery.
8. Zoe (57 years) needed skin surgery and was in hospital for three weeks.
9. Ed (70 years) needed surgery on his pancreas because he was in great pain. He was in hospital for three weeks at the time of the interview.
10. Al (67 years) had returned to hospital for more surgery when it was discovered that his cancer had recurred after the first operation.

Organization and layout of the themes

The qualitative themes that emerged from the interviews are organized and outlined below. Under the major heading, 'Patients experienced crushing vulnerability', several subthemes are described, which portray different aspects of the experience of crushing vulnerability. The following subthemes are some of the themes that characterize crushing vulnerability: (a) the hospital environment was strange; (b) anxiety about being treated like an object; (c) positive impact of being treated like a person; (d) shattering impact of cancer, and so on.

Finer discriminations may be found in some of these subthemes, so a third level of organization has occasionally been used. For example, in the subtheme (b) (anxiety about being treated like an object), the following subheadings have been used to identify different aspects of this subtheme: *ignored during the handovers*, and *public discussion of personal details was embarrassing*. An example of the organizing structure is represented in Box 6.1.

Box 6.1   Organization of the qualitative themes

Patients experienced crushing vulnerability (Level one, major theme, large/bold lettering)
(a) The hospital environment was strange (Level two, subtheme, alphabetically ordered)
(b) Anxiety about being treated like an object
    Ignored during handovers (Level three, very fine discrimination, italic lettering)
    Public discussion of personal details was embarrassing
(c) Positive impact of being treated like a person
(d) Shattering impact of cancer

Some word-for-word extracts from the interviews have been included in order to give a flavour of the interviews as a whole.

Theme 1: Patients experienced crushing vulnerability

Patients experienced being cared for at a time of crushing vulnerability. The emotional upheaval of being ill and in hospital was a particularly powerful emotional response.

(a) The hospital environment was strange

The hospital environment was experienced as a daunting place for a number of patients. This environment led some patients to become acutely aware of their own vulnerability and uncertainty about what they should do in this strange place. James, a 67-year-old retired headmaster, stated: 'I don't like being in a situation where I don't know what to do'.

Zoe was frightened and wondered what would happen to her. She had no control over her situation now, and had to rely on the staff. In hospital, strange people came to talk to her and to take blood samples. Other patients did not like being in hospital and were there because they had to be there – James was there 'under duress'.

Some patients were better able to cope with the hospital environment, especially those who had been hospital patients before, or who became accustomed to the place. However, this is not always true – one patient, Martha, spent several weeks in hospital after extensive plastic surgery. Although she knew the staff well and felt well cared for, she found herself crying from time to time because being in hospital just 'got to her'.

Being in hospital is a frightening experience. Patients are full of uncertainty and are unclear about what will happen to them. The unfamiliar surroundings heighten their inability to make predictions about even mundane aspects of their lives as patients. It is especially difficult to adapt to this environment at times of illness.

(b) Anxiety about being treated like an object

Nurses need to treat 'patients' as 'people'. The impersonal approach which staff employ in social interactions with patients can lead to anxiety. Some patients found that being in hospital induced anxiety about being *treated like an object*. Florence had a dreadful fear of being made to feel like a number. Similarly, James also expressed his own unease and said that he 'did not want to become just a name on a sheet of paper'.

This feeling can all too easily be created by staff in any hospital as they interact routinely with patients. Professionals regularly refer to people in hospital as 'patients', 'schizophrenics', 'diabetics', and so on, and this can all too easily degenerate into the type of non-person treatment that patients experience. We must remind ourselves constantly that the *patients are people*, too.

Patients try to deal with this anxiety. James was partially able to overcome being treated like an object by talking to other patients. Other patients were not so fortunate. Hugh's feelings were completely ignored by staff.

Ignored during the handovers

The handover between the different nursing shifts was usually conducted at the foot of Hugh's bed, and he was ignored by the staff. Hugh really wanted the nurses to talk *to* him, but instead the staff talked *about* him as if he did not exist: 'it's almost as if you're being talked about and are not there. You know "this is Mr D. who had a bath" . . . I'M HERE'.

Public discussion of personal details was embarrassing

During the staff handover at the bedside, the lack of privacy embarrassed Hugh: 'I don't think it should be done in front of the patient, being talked about is . . . embarrassing and wasted time'.

(c) Positive impact of being treated like a person

Some patients commented on the positive impact of being 'treated like a person'. It made them feel better and boosted their confidence.

Being treated like a person promoted recovery

Being treated like a person had a positive effect on some patients' well-being. It is widely acknowledged that psychological well-being can influence recovery rates (see, for example, Devine and Cook, 1983; Ley, 1988, Nichols, 1993). Although the staff did nothing dramatic for Florence, they did make her 'feel like a person, you know, not a number', and being treated like a person helped Florence to relax and to get better.

It felt good to be called by your first name

Some patients liked the staff to call them by their first name, but not every patient did. For some it appears to promote positive feelings, whereas for others it may promote unease and be interpreted as a lack of respect. One patient, Eileen, expressed the need for caution and felt that nurses should not call *all* patients by their first names; some patients, especially the older ones, do not like over-familiarity.

Staff did not make patients feel small

The positive attitude of the staff had an impact on patients, too. Staff did not make Florence feel 'small'; they were friendly and treated her like a workmate. Eileen felt that nurses would always respect her wishes, and that they would not take advantage of her. Tim had a very positive experience when he returned to the ward after going to another hospital for a series of diagnostic investigations. The nurses were genuinely glad to see him returning to the ward: 'When they seen me come back here last week, young Jane got hold of me as if she hadn't seen me for donkeys' years, as if I was a long-lost brother or something. They made me feel like somebody'.

(d) Shattering impact of cancer

Two of the informants in the study had recently been diagnosed as having cancer. This diagnosis had a tremendous impact on their lives and on their families.

Needed to know the truth

Both of the patients who developed cancer needed to know the truth about the condition and 'the future'. Tim needed to know 'the worst', but none of the doctors would tell him directly. This made him feel even more anxious about his condition and prognosis. When he was finally told he felt better, but he was very hurt because the doctor told his wife about the cancer before telling him. She was part of a 'conspiracy' and knew he had cancer when she came to visit him. Tim was kept in the dark and worried about the burden that had been placed on his wife's shoulders. Another patient, Al, asked the professor looking after him to tell him 'everything'.

Discovery

When Tim was eventually told he had lung cancer he went 'cold' and then he 'went to pieces'. Gradually he came to accept that he had cancer. Al's experience of cancer differed. In the beginning it all seemed like nothing – a small mole on his back which was eventually diagnosed as skin cancer. The professor told him he had cancer and that it was 'very serious'.

Thoughts about death and dying

Several patients spent time thinking about death and dying. When Al found out that he had terminal cancer he found himself in hospital thinking about his life: 'Life is sweet. I've got a little car, a wife and two nice children and we go and do things. Not a lot of money but it's nice. You know . . . after working all your life and retiring now comes the sallow days.'

Hope without guarantees

Patients wanted to have 'hope'. During his first operation, Al had a melanoma removed and the operation went well, but he knew that there were no guarantees, even though everything that could be done surgically had been done. Some time after the first operation another lump was discovered at out-patients, and a second operation was needed. The second operation went well, too. All he could do now was wait and see.

(e) Traumatic investigations and surgery

Lengthy and drawn out investigations were very traumatic for Tim. His condition was complicated by high blood pressure, and this meant that he had to move to another hospital for specialist care.

(f) Cancelled operation was a major setback

Tim's cancelled operation led him to assume that the cancer had spread to other parts of his body. He calmed down after hearing that the operation had not been cancelled altogether, but rather it was merely postponed until all of his test results were available.

(g) Anxious suspicion

Tim did not expect to be pampered, and felt that if he had been pampered or the nurses spent too much time with him, he would have suspected that something was seriously wrong: 'If they kept on I'm sure I'd think there was more wrong than is actually the case. That's how I would feel if they pampered me too much. I'd know. That I do believe.'

(h) Surrendering independence was distressing

Martha's lengthy stay in hospital was necessary because she needed a series of skin graft operations. She was in her thirties and found it hard to rely on other people and give up her independence. She felt clumsy at having to be helped to the toilet, and she was not able to sit up after the operations. It was very distressing and upsetting, especially after the second operation: 'I found it very difficult, very upsetting. I really thought that after six weeks I was going back to stage one.'

Gradually regained independence

Martha's independence was regained gradually, however. In the beginning the nurses had to do everything for her – washing, toileting, and changing positions, but they were able to judge what she could do for herself.

(i) Coping with bodily disfigurement was traumatic

Martha's operations involved skin grafting, and she found it very upsetting to look at the operation site and 'just to see it to start with was the worst bit, you feel like fainting'. However, she had to accept that she had a stoma, and she reached a point where she looked after herself independently.

(j) Difficulty in being away from home for a long time

Martha was away from her home and relatives for a long time, and her family could only visit her at weekends. Her GP told her that the surgery would take two or three weeks, but she had already spent eight weeks in hospital away from her family. Martha wanted staff to spend more time with her, but the staff were overly professional.

(k) Feeling like a smelly mess compared with the nurses

Zoe messed the floor because she had diarrhoea, and felt 'awful' because the student nurse had to clean it up. She compared herself to the nurses who were well groomed, while she felt like a 'smelly mess'.

(l) Feeling forgotten about

On one occasion Ed felt forgotten about because he had to wait five and a half hours for the doctor to come and set up an intravenous drip. He felt neglected, but at the same time Ed defended the staff by emphasizing how busy the nurses and doctors were: 'as I was saying there were other things doing and all. I don't suppose they can be in two places at once. But you're not the only one I expect there were others worse than I was like, that needed attending to.'

A brief comment on the theme

It should be clear that just arriving in hospital and settling into the routines to await an uncertain future is a complicated and anxiety-provoking experience. The physical environment, the technology, the uniformed staff and the specialist language used by the staff are all influential and contribute to the feeling of crushing vulnerability experienced by many if not all patients (Leigh and Reiser, 1980).

Some of the patients were ignored as people and their personal details were discussed in public during staff handovers, while other patients commented on the positive effect of being treated like a person while in hospital because it helped to promote recovery and made them feel good. The anxiety and vulnerability associated with being treated as an 'object' are discussed in detail by Van den Berg (1972), and are described by

Goffman (1968) as a type of 'non-person treatment' often found in the medical world.

Crushing vulnerability emphasizes each patient's need for sensitive nursing care. Inappropriate or tactless handling can have harmful psychological effects on the patient. Only one of the ten patients interviewed here was openly critical of the general care he received because he was made to feel like an 'object'. He had little say in his overall management, he was ignored during the handovers, his personal details were discussed publicly by the staff, and he had little contact with the trained staff. All these subtle and not so subtle actions made him feel like an object.

Theme 2: Patients adopted a particular mode of self-presentation

Several patients noted changes in their own behaviour that were linked to being ill and in hospital. They adopted particular modes of self-presentation consciously in some cases and without awareness in others. Some of the modes of presentation that were identified during the analysis of the interviews will now be described.

(a) Became sheepishly obedient

Some patients became very obedient. Florence did everything that the staff told her to do: 'Maybe I'm a bit sheepish'. She looked to doctors, nurses and other professionals when things went wrong because she had 'blind faith' in the professionals. James too was led by the needs of the staff, and made sure that he always gave staff the 'correct information'. He did not want to waste the staff's time, and he did what was asked of him unquestioningly.

Tim, an extremely nervous patient, met with many medical students because of his 'complicated and medically interesting' condition. However, it was not easy to be confronted by all of these powerful and professional people. Tim tolerated all the requests to be examined and probed because he felt that he would look foolish if he did not co-operate with the people who treated him. George was very co-operative during investigations, and removed his dressing gown and prepared himself 'patiently' on his bed for the different investigations.

(b) Conformed to the ritualistic practice

Another mode of self-presentation entailed conforming to ritualistic routines. George suggested that patients needed to abide by the ritualistic practice of the medicine round if the work was to get done. He was not 'allowed' to collect his medicine from the medicine trolley, but he did collect his own tea from the tea trolley.

(c) Became unusually friendly and cheerful

In a hospital there is suffering, pain and death all around the patients and staff. Some patients get better and are discharged, while others undergo a period of prolonged suffering and then die. Patients coped with the anxieties and uncertainties that the hospital aroused in different ways. One strategy was to adopt an unusually friendly and cheerful disposition. This is a strategy which is warmly welcomed by the staff. Several patients adopted a cheerfulness that was unfitting for the awful situations in which they found themselves – they felt obliged to try to be cheerful. However, one long-stay patient, Martha, described her stay as being as happy as it could have been in the circumstances.

(d) Provided a frank and honest account

One patient displayed an attitude of openness and honesty with staff which meant that they learned a great deal about him and his life while he knew nothing about them. This is a routine practice and the 'correct' way to proceed in a hospital context. Through this imbalance the patient's vulnerability is heightened while the power and status of the professional carer may be enhanced.

George told the truth about his excessive drinking. Not to tell the whole truth could damage his chances of recovery through inappropriate treatment. However, disclosing information about his drinking exposed him to the risk of being sanctioned or ignored by the staff like an unpopular patient, because conditions associated with 'drinking' may be regarded by the staff as being the patient's own fault.

(e) Helpful camaraderie amongst patients

Patients from different backgrounds and cultures are often thrown together by chance through the experience of illness. These people are drawn closer together both physically and psychologically because staff and the patients' relatives spend so little time with them. Patients often develop a comradeship amongst themselves to help and support each other – they make a point of helping each other.

Florence tried to help other patients to settle into the ward. Eileen did not need a lot of physical care, and had time to complete meal cards for the elderly patients and to help out at mealtimes. She only helped out so that the older patients were not left alone and unable to eat by themselves, and the staff appreciated her help. Al generally got on well with people and went around the ward and talked to other patients. The patients on the ward became pals.

The enforced camaraderie in the hospital ward obviously helps patients. It helps to reduce boredom and pass the time, as much of the patient's day is spent 'waiting'. These small groups are also likely to help patients to talk about their illness, investigations, treatments and so on as a way of dealing with anxiety, but some patients may find these informal conversations anxiety-provoking.

(f) Reluctant to ask questions

Patients were not encouraged to ask the staff questions, and this may be a characteristic part of the hospital culture. When patients did ask questions, the staff employed subtle tactics for letting them know that they should not make such enquiries – they let the patient know how busy they were, or gave the impression that the patient was being a nuisance, or provided incomplete answers to the patient's questions. These tactics had the effect of closing down any further communication.

Needed to keep up to date

Several patients needed more information. Some refrained from asking questions altogether, while others limited their enquiries to the sort of questions for which there was a simple 'yes' or 'no' answer. This meant that the questions did not make the staff feel uneasy and lead to upsetting situations. Patients were acutely aware of their lack of knowledge.

Did not want to bother the staff by asking questions

One way of ensuring that patients did not ask searching questions was to give the impression of 'busyness'. In the hospital culture, there is a tacit obligation to 'look busy', and this was obviously noted by some patients. The patients in this study were not encouraged to ask questions, although nobody actually told James *not to ask questions*. Hugh was made to feel like a nuisance for asking questions, especially by the doctors.

(g) Kept interpersonal encounters superficial

A number of patients kept their interpersonal encounters brief and superficial. James deliberately set limits on the interaction he had with others in the ward, and did not say a lot about his illness. He talked about superficial things like the weather, sport and television. More 'permanent relationships' were out of the question. Close relationships with nurses were not considered: 'It's me. That's the way I am, that's the way I've lived. I'm an ex-headmaster, I've had to learn to draw lines.'

George kept to himself and read; he did not go looking for conversations, but he talked constantly to his wife during visiting. Ed felt that the nurses did what they had to do and no more. They were not interested in or supposed to get closer to patients in hospital.

(h) Tried not to be a nuisance

Several patients tried not to be a 'nuisance'. James kept out of the way, especially when the staff were ill-tempered: 'they come on to a shift at seven in the morning after getting up at six and people can get up out of the wrong side of the bed. If you notice that, you know to keep your head down.'

When Ed was recovering and preparing to go home he just marched up and down the ward. Martha suggested that 'not being a nuisance' meant that other patients got their fair share of care and attention from the staff, but sometimes she was *made to feel guilty* by the staff who let her know that other patients on the ward needed looking after too.

(i) Provided a sense of purpose for the carers

Although in a very vulnerable position, some patients felt that they were able to give something back to the staff who cared for them, such as a sense of achievement. Zoe believed that seeing people get better gave nurses a sense of purpose. Not everyone felt this way.

(j) Showed deference and gratitude to the carers

Patients are generally very grateful for the care they receive. Al always displayed good manners and 'thanks' to the carers who looked after him. He really appreciated what was done for him and treated the staff respectfully.

(k) Admired the hard-working staff

There was much admiration for the work done by the staff for the patients in their care. Zoe could not understand how the nurses did some of the 'awful jobs' which they had to do, but she was very glad someone did them. Zoe, George and Florence suggested that the nurses were dedicated.

A brief comment on the theme

The patients adopted different roles in hospitalization. They needed to be perceived by the staff as people 'worthy' of care because they were vulnerable and in need of help. They also had to maintain their self-esteem. By fitting into the hospital environment and meeting the 'demand characteristics' of the situation, they could do this. A number of strategies of self-presentation were used by the patients. Some became sheepishly obedient or conformed to the ritualistic practices of the ward. Over-compliance can prove to be dangerous (see Ley, 1988).

Other patients became unusually cheerful and friendly in a situation that was terrifying and anxiety-provoking for them and probably for their relatives as well. These strategies of self-presentation are likely to be well received by the staff, and fit in well within the organizational culture. Cheerful, deferential and compliant patients are much more 'popular' than articulate, awkward and questioning patients (see Stockwell, 1972). People who work in hospitals tend to take the environment and all its 'trappings' for granted. Patients, relatives and others who are unfamiliar with the setting see it as an alien place and are often gripped by an uncertainty as to how to fit in. Conforming to the implicit and explicit demands of the staff is a 'safe' mode of self-presentation.

Some patients fitted in by providing a frank and honest account of their home and life circumstances. They made no attempt to cover up aspects of their lives which they might normally conceal in other social situations – they 'confessed' to the professional staff. The friendly camaraderie amongst the patients themselves was also found in another study by Coser (1962). In these small groups, patients had other people to talk to during the day and could exchange stories about their conditions, daily progress and things outside the hospital. However, when it came to asking questions of the staff patients were very reluctant. Coser (1962) also noted how new patients on a ward quickly learned 'what' to ask and 'what not' to ask, as well as 'who' to ask. Ley argued that patients' reluctance to ask questions stemmed 'mainly from over-deferential attitudes towards doctors' (Ley, 1988, p. 16).

In another research study, Waterworth and Luker (1990) emphasized the importance of 'toeing the line' as a patient. Showing admiration for the dedicated staff ensured that patients would be seen in a positive light by the staff. These self-presentation 'tactics' helped patients to cope with anxiety.

Theme 3: Patients evaluated the hospital services

Patients' evaluations of the hospital services were generally positive, but there were instances in which patients were critical of the staff and the organization.

(a) General level of satisfaction with the caring staff

There was a general level of satisfaction with the care received, and many patients genuinely appreciated what was being done for them. As consumers, they were satisfied with the level of care. The technical facets of the nurses' role were primary. Ed felt that hospital was the best place for him because there was nobody to look after him at home. James found that the staff in other hospitals were not so caring, while the staff here were excellent. Florence knew that the staff were 'doing their best' for her.

Limited but satisfactory level of nursing care

The level of contact between the professional carers and the patients did appear to be very limited. Not every patient had a lot of nursing attention; some did not have any 'real' nursing (basic/physical nursing care), only 'tests' such as chest X-rays, and blood and urine investigations. These patients were described by the staff as 'self-caring', and they received only a very limited amount of nursing time. However, some of the patients felt that 'staff let the patients know they were there for them if they really needed them'.

Because some of the patients did not need a lot of physical care, the contact with the nurses was limited to the times when the nurses had to perform routines that were completed quickly. The limited contact between the nurses and some of the patients could mean that psychological care of patients was lacking in this context. Physical care often presents the nurse with an opportunity for 'talking' to the patient and exploring that patient's personal view of the world.

High levels of nursing care needed

Other patients needed a lot of physical care. Zoe had to be helped in and out of the bath initially and then she had to be helped to walk. Gradually she became more independent and needed less help from the nurses. There was evidence here that the staff provided very thoughtful nursing and tried to prevent over-dependence. In the beginning the nurses had to do everything for Zoe. As time passed they let Zoe dress herself as soon as it was feasible for her to do so. Martha was very dependent immediately after her operation.

(b) Staff were friendly but diplomatic

Although the contact between patients and nursing staff was limited, several patients commented on the positive effect of having 'friendly' staff around them. The informal and friendly atmosphere was helpful. Zoe also commented on the friendliness of the staff, but she noted how 'careful' and 'diplomatic' the staff were when talking about her illness.

(c) Nurses asked what the patients needed

Martha was confined to bed for some time and without frequent visitors. Most of the nurses asked if she needed washing or shopping to be done. One young student nurse took Marth's dressing gown home overnight and washed it for her. Others brought in magazines for her to look at to help pass the time and alleviate boredom.

(d) Felt safe and trusted the nurses

The nurses had to do a lot for Martha, and she trusted them and felt at ease with them. She felt safe because they held her firmly when she had to get into the bath, although some nurses made her feel safer than others.

(e) Technical competence was appreciated

Many patients praised the skill and expertise that characterized the nurses' performance. Injections were administered competently and sensitively, and blood samples were taken speedily and skilfully. Staff also ensured that medicines were given on time. The experienced nurses were good at handling drips, dressings, etc. although this was not always true of less experienced nurses. Nurses made constant checks on the patients and responded promptly when someone rang a call bell. The nurses were perceived by the patients to be 'always on their toes' and it was felt that they 'earned their money'. It was clear that all of the patients evaluated the performance of the staff and recognized more competent behaviour.

(f) The approach of the staff was sensitive and calming

The nurses' ability to calm Tim when he was a very anxious patient, without resorting to the use of minor tranquillizers, was important. When Al came into hospital he was very apprehensive, but the staff quickly dispelled any fears that he had.

Watched the carers in action from a distance

Patients become observers of the way in which staff manage other patients. George watched the nurses and doctors in action from a distance. He could not help overhearing things as the nurses calmed a very frightened patient. The nurses just sat with the frightened patient and quickly arranged for a social worker to help the patient's wife, who was alone and disabled.

Aware that the nurses understood her loneliness

When Martha's husband came to visit her at the weekend the nurses gave her husband a spare meal so that he could stay with her and would not have to go down to the canteen, which was some distance from the ward. The nurses knew that he had to travel a long distance to be with his wife and that in a few short hours he would have to travel home to look after Martha's sick mother. This 'bending of the rules' by the nurses had a big impact on the way Martha perceived the nursing staff. She knew that they understood her loneliness.

(g) The accommodation and hotel services were reasonable

Several patients mentioned the importance of accommodation and hotel services during their stay in hospital. In general, the quality of the food was good, and the bed linen was changed daily. However, one patient noted that the china was cracked and ought to have been replaced. Zoe found the hospital clean.

(h) The devoted student nurses were constantly available

The student nurses were singled out by several patients for their attentive care and devotion. The younger nurses were always available. None of the patients objected to the fact that they were looked after mainly by student nurses rather than trained and more experienced nurses, because these young nurses had to gain experience in order to fulfil their training requirements. The 'constant availability' of the students was very notable and much appreciated.

The students took time and talked

Students spent more time with the patients and got to know them better than the qualified staff. Some of the experienced students were very used to talking with patients and were very good at it. The students took time to talk to patients and shared 'a bit of their lives' – they did not simply collect information from the patients and give nothing back.

The students listened and tried to answer questions

Talking to the students helped to keep Hugh's spirits up, because they were very helpful. They 'listened' attentively to him and tried to answer his questions. Occasionally they tried to answer questions beyond the level of their experience and knowledge.

Appreciated the students who stayed late

Martha really appreciated one of the students who stayed on late to complete her care even though her shift had finished and other members of staff had gone home. The student did not want the new night shift to come in before she had finished settling Martha down for the night.

Students went around with the doctors

Not all of the patients were particularly appreciative of the students' approach. Ed, who had little contact with students, noted how they went around with the doctors. It was just as he had expected it to be in hospital. In general the staff tended to ignore him.

(i) Helped to get through the miserable nights

Several patients mentioned that the nights were difficult. It was a time that Zoe found particularly hard because she could not sleep well. She found herself tired but restless at night, and it was unpleasant to be woken up so early in the morning when she wanted a lie-in, but she had to fit in with the ward routine. Several patients commented that other patients coughing during the night disrupted their sleep. However, some patients found the night staff very helpful because they made tea during the night to help patients sleep – just as they would do at home. The night staff were also pleased to see Zoe and asked how she was 'getting on' after they returned from their nights off. They told her how well her wound was healing, and they reassured her about her progress.

(j) Did not get to know nurses well

It is often claimed that the relationship between patients and nurses is the foundation for providing good nursing care. It was notable that patients did not get to know any of the nurses. Contact between patients and nurses was often limited to 'tablet time'. Nevertheless, some patients did not see a need to get to know the nurses well. They just wanted to be looked after by competent staff who treated them like 'people'. Patients did see a lot more of the students and unqualified nursing staff because they came around regularly to perform basic care and make observations.

Minimal contact with qualified staff

Unlike the student group, the trained nurses spent even less time interacting with the patients. Surprisingly, Hugh did not even speak to the ward sister at any time during his admission. This was not the case on other wards where he had been a patient. The lack of contact with trained staff made a big difference to the patients' day. One of the patients observed how on one ward the qualified staff *found* things for the students to do if they saw them talking to patients or sitting down at the patient's bedside.

Superficial contact with trained nurses

When contact *was* established with the trained nursing staff it tended to be rather superficial. George just passed the time of day with staff by talking about the weather, television, the most recent news items, and so on. Some interactions with patients were limited to the nurse asking a patient to get off his or her bed so that it could be made up.

The staff were awfully busy

Patients generally perceived the staff as being 'too busy' to talk to them, or else they felt that other seriously ill patients needed attention more urgently.

Several patients commented that the nurses were too busy and did not have time to talk: 'The nurses didn't talk about the operation because they're awfully busy, they'll talk to you – yes. "How are you today? How's your wound? Let's have a look at it, that's fine, that's coming on nicely". That sort of thing. But I mean they are awfully busy and there is a lot of physical work attached.'

It was suggested that the really ill patients needed a lot of attention and rest and that the staff had to get on with their difficult work. It was also suggested that staff movements (shift patterns, staff reallocations, and students' placements) were responsible for the lack of time available to be with the patients. Other patients were not bothered by staff movements and accepted the lack of interaction with the staff as a feature of the system of hospital care. Another patient felt that some staff *gave the impression* of being understaffed, while others were always relaxed and ensured that patients were well cared for no matter what pressure they were under.

(k) Nothing was too much trouble

The attitude of the caring nurses was captured by several patients in this subtheme. Zoe felt that the staff were genuinely busy but they still gave the impression that 'nothing was too much trouble'. They got the phone for her on many occasions and placed it beside her bed so that she could phone home. Paying attention to small details can make a big difference to the quality of care that patients experience. The 'nothing was too much trouble' attitude was mentioned by several patients.

(l) No front – just genuine nurses

Tim commented that there was no 'front' to the nurses' attitude, and that they always displayed a concern 'for his well-being' and it was a genuine concern. Hugh described the approach of the students as genuine and not patronizing – but the qualified nurses were different.

(m) Displayed a caring attitude in their work

The nurses had time for the 'personal touch' which was important for George – he described this as a 'caring attitude', and it showed in the way that the nurses looked after the patients on the ward.

(n) The doctors were approachable

Some doctors, too, were singled out for comment; the doctors were 'good and introduced themselves' to the patients when they came to the bedside. This made them seem more human and less frightening. The doctors allowed Florence to ask questions and she felt more confident when she did so. Another patient felt that the doctors were 'exceptional'.

(o) Key criticisms of the staff

Several important criticisms of the staff also emerged, and these highlighted the need for staff to listen carefully to what patients have to say. This is an important step in meeting the needs of patients as consumers.

Rude staff

The importance of good manners was highlighted. George commented on the rude tea ladies – one of whom 'almost threw the tea' at him, and the auxiliary nurse, who was particularly rude. Zoe had an upsetting argument with a rude receptionist about her special diet, and she became very upset and very angry about the whole incident, which could easily have been avoided.

Hurried approach of the nurses provoked anxiety

Martha needed extensive nursing care after her operations and she did not like it when the nurses were 'in a rush' – especially when she was in pain. Being rushed made her feel 'on edge' and the nurses tended to 'dash through their work' when they were short of staff. Zoe needed regular baths, and noticed that the busy auxiliaries were constantly trying to get her into the bath in a 'hurried' fashion.

Kept in the dark

Some patients were not given enough information about their illness and treatment. There was a general lack of information on some wards; patients sometimes even had to ask what their tablets were for. Hugh did not like to take the tablets unless he knew exactly what they were for. Several patients were not told why certain things were done, and that strategy seemed routine: 'there's a definite lack of information. They do things but you don't know why half of the time'.

   One patient suggested that the staff were 'trained to keep people in the dark'. The blame for not informing patients was placed firmly with the doctors and nurses by the patients who felt let down by the lack of information. The nurses and doctors were seen as the people responsible for telling people about illness, treatment, investigations and management.

Boredom

Boredom is a common feature of patients' experience. Hospital became boring for Zoe, but there were no organized activities on the ward. She was left to 'entertain' herself by whatever means she could during the day. This meant that most patients were left to 'wait' and to think about what might happen to them.

Poor nursing practice

Eileen observed what she described as poor nursing practice. The staff gave the elderly patients far too much food at mealtimes. Many of the older patients ate very slowly, and some did not have their dentures in place during the meals. The large portions of food were not suitable for old people. Eileen filled in the meal cards for the elderly patients who were unable to do this for themselves, and she ordered smaller portions on the meal cards without consulting the nurses, who had not noticed this problem.

A brief comment on the theme

It was difficult to see how these vulnerable patients could have been critical of a system that, along with serious illness, made them so dependent. Their attention was focused on things that may have seemed unimportant to the staff. The friendliness of the staff was significant to patients. The fact that the staff bothered to ask patients what they needed, and their ability to make the patients feel safe, influenced the patients' opinions greatly. The technical competence of the staff in giving injections and other procedures was much appreciated, too. All of these issues are simple components of the nurses' daily work, and they contributed to the positive perceptions of the staff by the patients. It was clear that many members of staff were good at the job of caring for patients.

It has been suggested that the routine 'services' greatly influence patients' perceptions of care and the expressed level of satisfaction with services (Rempusheski *et al.*, 1988). Patients were generally satisfied with the care that they received, although some very pointed criticisms were made. These could so easily have been put right with careful planning, and perhaps some additional training.

It is clear that some nurses pay little or no attention to patients' diet. While this may seem reasonable to some, because of changes in the way that hotel services are delivered, it ignores the importance that the patients place on these 'hotel' facilities. Having clean bed linen, or a clean and uncracked cup to drink out of, have symbolic meaning for the patients. They may convey to the patient a message that he or she is a *person worthy of care*, and not an object.

The student nurses and the night staff were singled out for praise, but the qualified and more senior nursing staff may need to think carefully about their role. Are they providers of direct patient care or managers of such services? The trained staff were generally perceived by patients as being too busy. This finding is consistent with the general tendency for much of the basic nursing to be done by the learners in particular, or by untrained staff (Knight and Field, 1981; Robinson *et al.*, 1989).

Patients are usually very reluctant to voice any criticism of the staff to anyone remotely involved with the system. This may be the result of an implicit rule of being a vulnerable patient – one must never criticize, for criticism is likely to lead to patients being labelled either 'good' or 'bad' (Lorber, 1975; Kelly and May, 1982) or unpopular (Stockwell, 1972), and treated accordingly. It is notable that most of the official complaints about hospital highlight 'poor communication' as the major source of patient dissatisfaction. It is also notable that the number of official complaints about care has increased rapidly in recent years (Audit Commission, 1993).

Theme 4: Patients' personal concerns assumed great importance

The patients' personal concerns are not always recognized by the staff, yet they are important for patients. The personal concerns of patients may influence the patients' perceptions of the context in which care is experienced. However, the personal concerns mentioned here cannot reflect the concerns of *all* patients. The issues raised give only a flavour of the sorts of things that are a focus for patients' thoughts and feelings. These may be a constant source of patient anxiety, and may go unnoticed by staff.

(a) The treatment was primary

Many patients felt that the *treatment* was the most important aspect of being in hospital. Patients may perceive the nurse's role as primarily one of ensuring that patients get the right treatment. This was certainly the case with James, who was only concerned about his treatment – nothing else mattered to him. Similarly, Ed just needed an operation to put things right, and then he could get out of the hospital and resume his normal life outside.

Nurses can also make an effort to improve the quality of *that individual's care* by being well informed about his or her treatment and medical management, and ensuring that he or she is kept up to date. The importance of the nurse's role in giving information to patients and their relatives has been widely demonstrated (see, for example, Devine and Cook, 1983).

(b) Being in hospital was frustrating

Being in hospital can be a very frustrating time for patients. The patient's whole life has been altered by illness, and his or her work, social life and personal relationships have been seriously disrupted. In some cases, such as life-threatening illness, unexpected trauma, or the diagnosis of a stigmatizing illness such as breast cancer or schizophrenia, a person's life may be ruined. While some patients may be in hospital for investigations and are obviously not acutely 'ill', others may be there for life-saving surgery, to have children, or for more long-term treatment.

Frustration can arise from different sources. The fact that a person's life is temporarily disrupted may be bad enough, but having to ask a nurse for a 'bottle' may be embarrassing and frustrating, too. Hugh was disheartened because he felt pretty well in himself, but he *had to stay in bed*. Using a commode beside the bed in a ward with other patients may be particularly anxiety-provoking. Many patients in hospital may be able to look after themselves. They are often referred to as 'self-caring' during the daily report, because they do not need much direct nursing. Yet these individuals are often subject to the same restrictive regimes that many acutely ill patients willingly undergo without question.

(c) Felt let down by the GP after husband's death

During her interview Florence talked a lot about her GP, who was very supportive when her husband died. He was one of those doctors who was 'always available and willing to talk' to her about the death of her husband and her own health. Since her husband had died, Florence too had become ill and needed to make more frequent calls on the GP service. As time went by, Florence began to feel 'neglected' and 'let down' by the GP and his colleagues, who lacked patience. Eventually Florence did see the consultant surgeon, and this led to her admission to hospital for surgery.

(d) Mother's recent death

Eileen recounted how her mother had died recently, just before she had to come into hospital. Eileen had had to deal with the death, the funeral and its aftermath, and this experience continued to play a very significant part in her life, even though she now found herself in hospital and in need of treatment.

This is a particularly good example of the nurses' need to take account of the important things that may be happening or have recently happened to a person who arrives on the ward as a patient. People who are bereaved usually need to talk to others about the bereavement, which enters every aspect of a person's life, and may be thought about constantly. Nurses may need to set aside time to talk to the patient, and this background material will help them to meet a particular patient's needs and to draw up an appropriate plan of care. However, this is difficult to do, and it is anxiety-provoking for some nurses. In addition, it may cause some conflict between colleagues who may have a more 'detached' approach to patients (see Menzies, 1970).

(e) The previous admission to hospital was terrible

Nurses often forget that many patients may have a 'patient career' which can span several years and numerous admissions. Previous admissions can help the patient to come into hospital in a more settled state of mind, but they can also generate crippling anxiety. One patient, George, described his previous admission to hospital for major surgery for a damaged kidney. It was a very disappointing experience. He was discharged before he had made a full recovery because the hospital needed to vacate beds for new patients awaiting admission.

(f) Concerned about the family and close friends

The final topic to emerge as an important aspect of the patients' personal concerns dealt with their families and friends. At times of illness, people obtain physical and psychological support from other family members. These family members, friends, or partners may provide different forms of social support for patients. For many patients such supporting mechanisms work very well. Unfortunately, other patients do not have this type of support, and may themselves be the major supportive force in the lives of others outside the hospital.

Professional helpers naturally enough often see the patient as *the* member of the family who is in crisis. Some patients, however, may be especially concerned about the health and well-being of the other family members who are *not* in hospital. Martha's mother, for example, lived over 250 miles away from the hospital, and herself needed an operation to save the sight in her one good eye. She needed her daughter to look after her, but Martha was stranded in hospital with no chance of a speedy recovery and discharge. Martha's mother and her husband were all the family she had, and being far away from them was a 'constant source of worry'.

Another elderly patient, Ed, was very concerned about the one 'visitor' who came to see him every day. She had to travel to the hospital by public transport, and this meant she had to change buses twice, and it took her over an hour to get to the hospital. It was a long way for an elderly person to travel, and the travelling took up much of her day. Ed was grateful that she came to see him, but he was 'worried about her health' because she had arthritis in her leg and was 'not very good on her feet'. She found it very difficult to get around, and waiting for buses in bad weather was not good for her.

In the busy hospital environment these personal concerns for others outside hospital may often go unrecognized by nurses and doctors. Not every patient had to deal with these 'personal concerns', but for those who did, they were very real sources of anxiety and uncertainty.

A brief comment on the theme

This theme emphasized more details about the patients' experiences that were very personal. These issues may go unnoticed by the staff. However, the personal concerns of the patients served as important reminders of life outside hospital and the need for patients to continue to deal with issues and relationships outside, and nurses need to set aside time to learn about these personal concerns. Staff may be able to offer support and, where appropriate, practical help. Training in the approach used to guide the interviews and the analysis of these may be a useful starting point.

Important issues in the nurse/patient relationship

In this section some of the wider issues that may influence the nurse/patient relationship are discussed. The relationship between patients and nurses is complex. The patient enters into the relationship through illness, while nurses and other health-care workers are there to help as professionals.

Power

The issue of 'power' in the nurse/patient relationship is important because it may cast a shadow over what nurses do. Morse (1991) reported a research study in which interviews with 86 nurses were analysed using the grounded theory approach. The idea of 'negotiating the relationship' between the patient and the nurse emerged as an important item and this meant 'involvement' and 'commitment'. However, Morse did not mention the fact that any form of negotiation must occur from different perspectives. If the perspectives were the same, there would be no need to negotiate.

The scenario described in this chapter illustrates how the patient is in a *very vulnerable* position, while the nurse is in a position of *control and power*. These different positions are clearly highlighted in the study outlined here, but they have also been recognized in other studies involving patients (see, for example, Robinson, 1968; May, 1990). The impact of the status and social position of the individuals participating in these negotiations must be more fully understood if we are to develop helpful relationships with patients. Guggenbühl-Craig's (1971) analysis of professional carers (therapists, doctors and social workers) revealed a *desire for power over clients* amongst these professional groups.

Clearly nurses also hold power over patients, and the desire for 'nursing' to become more 'professional' can only increase this power. Great care is needed if we are to develop and enhance patient care. Nurses should not forget that their primary role is to look after patients. Professional developments in education and research are important, but they must be guided by the need to improve direct care in different areas.

The ideal of mutuality

The concept of mutuality is closely related to the power issue. Rogers (1967) suggested that the relationship between the one being helped and the helper *is a mutual one* in therapy, but this is a contentious viewpoint. The goal of mutuality is more an ideal state that cannot be achieved in a professional helping context. The philosopher Martin Buber (1966) suggested that, because the patient comes to the professional for help, the relationship can *never be a mutual one:*

> He comes for help to you. You don't come for help to him. And not only this, but you are *able*, more or less, to help him. He can do different things to you, but not help you. . . . You are, of course, a very important person for him. But not a person whom he wants to see and to know and is able to. . . . He is, may I say, entangled in your life, in your thoughts, in your being, your communication, and so on. But he is not interested in you as you. It cannot be. You are interested in . . . him as this person. This kind of detached presence he cannot have and give.
>
> (Buber, 1966, p. 171)

It is difficult to see how 'mutuality' could be achieved in practice, except in cases where a long-term relationship between the patient and the nurse has developed and has been maintained over time.

The importance of physical care

The importance of the physical/basic care of the patient must not be overlooked. There is an obvious and *crucial link* between physical and psychological nursing care, because the need to complete basic care tasks means that a nurse *must spend time with a patient*. This time presents the nurse with an opportunity to interact with the patient while completing this basic care. Paradoxically, basic care is often provided by untrained nurses and students – the least well-trained staff have the closest contact with patients. Psychological care of patients is not closely linked with the provision of basic nursing care by trained and experienced staff. In another research study of medical and surgical nurses in a German hospital, a similar picture emerged (Morrison and Bauer, 1993), while Smith stated that:

> The patient makes clear links between the emotional and physical aspects of her care. She describes caring gestures, the little things that make her feel qualitatively different: nurses who recognised she needed to talk, were good listeners, held her hand, took away her fear and had a calming influence on her. She described them as 'brilliant', indicating that she recognised they had skills, but also implied that these caring gestures were 'natural'. . . . Emotional labour does make a difference, and care matters to patients, but it is still in danger of being marginalised.
>
> (Smith, 1992, p. 145)

Patients also need technically competent nurses and doctors to look after them. There is a need for balance between the necessity for good technical, basic care and psychological care.

When nurses provide direct physical or basic care (and to a lesser extent technical care), they are provided with a *bridge* for giving psychological care to the patient. Trained practising nurses themselves recognize this, but continue to emphasize the 'managerial' aspects of the role that assume greater importance within the organizational hierarchy and culture (Morrison, 1991, 1992). Trained nurses need to refocus on the link between the physical and psychological care of the patient in order to provide individualized care for the patient.

There is also a need for managers of nursing services to address the issue of the psychological care of patients. The stated aim of most nursing units is to provide 'quality care', and that includes physical and psychological aspects of care. Clearly, time is needed to build good relationships. If more trained nurses are to become involved in direct patient care, then managers must take account of that fact and begin to change the culture of organizations so that basic care is not seen as low-status work to be left to the untrained staff.

Ordinary patients and ordinary nurses

There is a great emphasis in the current literature on psychological care of the patient. The positive effects of being an *ordinary person* who happens to be a nurse helping other ordinary people should not be underestimated. Patients need to know that those looking after them are human, too. In a study of 'informal' helping, Cowen (1982) described how members of the public sought help from different occupational groups. The study examined peoples' willingness to discuss 'psychological problems', such as difficulties with children, job insecurity, loneliness, problems with colleagues and depression, with hairdressers, lawyers, supervisors and bartenders, rather than seeking out an expert in mental health.

The informal helpers offered a wide range of helpful interventions – they offered support and sympathy, tried to make light of the problems, listened, offered alternative solutions, shared their personal experiences, gave advice, asked questions, and pointed out the consequences of bad ideas or tried to get the person to talk to someone else. All the groups generally felt good about offering this very 'ordinary' service to customers and believed themselves to be moderately good at it. Nurses should try to develop this 'ordinary' and 'spontaneous' approach in nursing practice.

Kleinman (1988) argued that professional socialization produced doctors that he referred to as 'disabled' healers:

> Professional training, in principle then, should make it feasible for practitioners to deliver care that is both technically competent and humane, whether or not

they are personally motivated toward a particular patient or work under threatening conditions. Certain aspects of professional training seem to disable practitioners. The professional mask may protect the individual practitioner from feelings of being overwhelmed by patients' demands, but it may also cut him off from the human experience of illness.

(Kleinman, 1988, p. 225)

A very similar training pattern can be seen in the nursing profession (see Menzies, 1970). In truth, very little attention is paid to the human component of nursing work.

If the implicit desire within the profession is to 'care for people', that means having contact with people who happen to be ill, and this desire is built upon a natural helping attitude which many learners bring with them to the job, then this attitude needs to be fostered during a period of socialization. For this to happen, learners need good role models and a supportive learning environment (Pratt, 1980). It is the responsibility of practitioners, as well as the teaching, administrative and policy-making staff, to ensure that these requirements are not overlooked *if* we really want to emphasize the psychological side of the nursing role.

Conclusions

The detailed account of patients' experiences of being cared for in hospital emphasizes the need for high-quality nursing care of patients. The issues to emerge here will help practitioners to reflect carefully on their own approach to patients and their families. An in-depth insight into patients' experiences is needed if nurses are to develop a sound understanding of patients and to provide care that is both appropriate and effective.

References

Audit Commission (1993) *What Seems To Be The Matter? Communication Between Hospitals And Patients*. HMSO, London.

Buber M (1966) *The Knowledge of Man: a Philosophy of the Interhuman* (transl. by Friedman M and Smith RG). Harper and Row, New York.

Coser RL (1962) *Life in the Ward*. Michigan State University, Michigan.

Cowen EL (1982) Help where you find it. Four informal helping groups. *American Psychologist* 37, 385–95.

Devine EC and Cook TD (1983) A meta-analytical analysis of effects of psycho-educational interventions on length of post-surgical surgical hospital stay. *Nursing Research* 32, 267–74.

Goffman E (1968) *Asylums: Essays on the Social Situation of Mental Patients and Other Inmates*. Penguin, Harmondsworth.

Guggenbühl-Craig A (1971) *Power in the Helping Professions*. Spring, University of Dallas, Irving.

Kelly MP and May P (1982) Good and bad patients: a review of the literature and a theoretical critique. *Journal of Advanced Nursing* 7, 147–56.

Kestenbaum V (ed.) (1982) *The Humanity of the Ill: Phenomenological Perspectives.* University of Tennessee Press, Knoxville.

Kleinman A (1988) *The Illness Narratives: Suffering, Healing and the Human Condition.* Basic Books, New York.

Knight M and Field D (1981) Silent conspiracy: coping with dying cancer patients on acute surgical wards. *Journal of Advanced Nursing* 6, 221–9.

Leigh H and Reiser ME (1980) *The Patient. Biological, Psychological, and Social Dimensions of Medical Practice.* Plenum, New York.

Ley P (1988) *Communicating with Patients: Improving Communication, Satisfaction and Compliance.* Chapman and Hall, London.

Lorber J (1975) Good patients and problem patients: conformity and deviance in a general hospital. *Journal of Health and Social Behaviour* 16, 213–25.

May C (1990) Research on nurse–patient relationships: problems of theory, problems of practice. *Journal of Advanced Nursing* 15, 307–15.

Menzies IEP (1970) *The Functioning of Social Systems as a Defence Against Anxiety.* Centre for Applied Social Research, Tavistock Institute of Human Relations, London.

Morrison P (1991) *The Meaning of Caring Interpersonal Relationships in Nursing.* PhD thesis, Sheffield Hallam University, Sheffield.

Morrison P (1992) *Professional Caring in Practice. A Psychological Analysis.* Avebury, Aldershot.

Morrison P (1994) *Understanding Patients.* Balliere Tindall, London.

Morrison P and Bauer I (1993) A clinical application of the multiple sorting technique. *International Journal of Nursing Studies* 30, 511–18.

Morse JM (1991) Negotiating commitment and involvement in the nurse–patient relationship. *Journal of Advanced Nursing* 16, 455–68.

Nicholls KA (1993) *Psychological Care in Physical Illness*, 2nd edn. Chapman and Hall, London.

Pratt R (1980) A time to every purpose … *The Australian Nurses' Journal* 10, 50–6.

Rempusheski VF, Chamberlain SL, Picard HB, Ruzanski J and Collier M (1988) Expected and received care: patient perceptions. *Nursing Administration Quarterly* 12, 42–50.

Robinson L (1968) *Psychological Aspects of the Care of Hospitalised Patients.* FA Davis, Philadelphia.

Robinson J, Stilwell J, Hawley C and Hempstead N (1989) *The Role of the Support Worker in the Ward Health Care Team.* Nursing Policy Studies Centre and Health Service Unit, University of Warwick.

Rogers CR (1967) *On Becoming a Person: a Therapist's View of Psychotherapy.* Constable, London.

Smith P (1992) *The Emotional Labour of Nursing. Its Impact on Interpersonal Relations, Management and the Educational Environment in Nursing.* Macmillan, London.

Stevenson L (1987) *Seven Theories of Human Nature*, 2nd edn. Oxford University Press, Oxford.

Stockwell F (1972) *The Unpopular Patient.* Royal College of Nursing, London.

Taylor SJ and Bogdan R (1984) *Introduction to Qualitative Research Methods. The Search for Meanings*, 2nd edn. Wiley, New York.

Van den Berg JH (1972) *The Psychology of the Sickbed.* Humanities Press, New York.

Waterworth S and Luker K (1990) Reluctant collaborators: do patients want to be involved in decisions concerning care? *Journal of Advanced Nursing* 15, 971–6.

Further reading

Audit Commission (1993) *What Seems to the Matter? Communication Between Hospitals and Patients.* HMSO, London.

Morrison P (1991) *Professional Caring in Practice: A Psychological Analysis.* Avebury Press, Aldershot.

Morrison P and Burnard P (1991) *Caring and Communicating: The Interpersonal Relationship in Nursing.* Macmillan Press, Basingstoke.

Acknowledgement

Thanks are due to Ballière Tindall for permission to reproduce a shortened account of some material that appeared in Morrison P (1994) *Understanding patients.*

7

Reflecting on ritual: an anthropological approach to personal rituals and care among Gujarati women in east London

Meg McDonald

Before a nurse ever encounters a patient or client, 'the patient' has already developed a culturally appropriate and personally significant approach to daily living. Our daily living, in health and disease, and through good times and sorrow and anxieties, is circumscribed by ritual and punctuated by cultural norms. In our multi-ethnic society it is not possible to understand or become acquainted with all the customs and traditions of the people we may encounter. The significance for nurses, as Leininger observed in the 1970s and nurse anthropologists are still confirming today, is that there are many ways of demonstrating care, and that care is an important human quality cross-culturally. There is no culture without forms of recognizable and deliberate caring acts of compassion and concern, and this includes care at times of illness and vulnerability. This chapter looks at formal and informal caring rituals among one ethnic group that UK nurses may encounter, namely Gujarati women. Their wise and compassionate care is steeped in a different tradition to that of most European nurses, but is none the less a wonderful reflection of the healing and unifying power of culture. It is a reminder of the power of culture in our lives, and the comforting familiarity of rituals and caring practices. The better we understand and appreciate our culture, the better we understand and appreciate ourselves.

Introduction

For several years, nurses have increasingly been recognizing that caring involves an understanding of the way in which culture informs experiences of health and illness. Nurses are also becoming increasingly aware of the potential of anthropology in contributing to a greater understanding of human cultural diversity. Anthropology and nursing share several common features: both are concerned with a holistic approach; both focus on human relationships; and both disciplines recognize reflection as a means of increasing self-knowledge and awareness. For anthropologists, such self-knowledge comes from cross-cultural comparison which challenges our own assumptions and Western presuppositions. Michael Carrithers makes this point well:

> Socrates urged that we reflect on ourselves (he said 'the unexamined life is not worth living'); anthropologists would insist that such reflection include a mutual, shared life as well.
>
> (Carrithers, 1992, p. 1)

Crucially, he goes on to note that 'we cannot know each other except by knowing ourselves in relation to others' (ibid.). The focus of anthropology is not 'other' exotic non-Western cultures for, as Ingold (1992) cogently points out, in anthropology we study ourselves. The 'we' he refers to is the inclusive global nature of human life.

With this reflexive challenge in mind, the present chapter attempts to elucidate a particular aspect of caring which has received little attention in the nursing literature, namely the promotion of health and well-being through ritual. It describes the personal rituals which Gujarati women in east London enact in order to care for members of their household and family. More than this, it suggests that reflecting on these rituals provides useful insights into the cultural construction of nursing knowledge and practice, enabling us to know and better understand the way in which we care. The first section examines reflexivity from an anthropological perspective, and then goes on to discuss the way in which ritual is understood in both nursing and anthropology. Ethnographic data based on fieldwork in east London are used to examine personal rituals and care among Gujarati women. It is suggested that, in reflecting on these rituals, several concepts emerge which are salient to nursing care and practice.

Reflexivity in nursing and anthropology

Nursing and anthropology share a particular focus on reflection, or reflexivity as it is known in anthropology. Similarities exist in the use of these terms in that there is an emphasis in both disciplines on self-knowledge and critical awareness. Nursing is especially concerned with a gradual process of self-awareness and critical appraisal of action which results in a growth of knowledge and competence (Powell, 1989; Coutts-Jarman, 1993; Atkins and Murphy, 1993). To a large extent, nursing theories of reflection are informed by educational theorists (Dewey, 1933; Schon, 1983; Boud *et al.*, 1985; Jarvis, 1992), and reflection in nursing is often linked to learning contexts (Palmer *et al.*, 1994). While Fitzgerald (1994) also identifies a literature which focuses on a critical inquiry of nursing, both as a discipline itself and in relation to the wider fabric of society (Salvage, 1985; Street, 1992), this aspect is not usually included in discussions of reflection in nursing.

In anthropology, reflexivity is also part of a wider discourse which has developed with post-modernist, and especially feminist (Caplan, 1988), theory. Scholte (1972) was an early exponent, and in a critique of the ideology of a value-free social science, he noted two strands to reflexivity: the self-reflecting anthropologist as he or she goes about ethnographic research, and a broader approach to the discipline itself – a questioning of the way in which anthropologists accumulate knowledge about other cultures. The former strand entails a recognition of the self, including one's own culture and gender, and the way in which this impinges on the fieldwork process. Okely (1992, p. 3) describes this process as one which 'is totalising and draws on the whole being'. The latter strand has become known as the 'politics of representation' – how it is that our own Western biases and presuppositions shape the way in which we 'know' others and interpret what it is they say and do. As Cornwall and Lindisfarne have observed:

> A basic precept of anthropological studies is that new insights into social relations follow the investigation of cultural categories that have previously been taken for granted. . . . New, and often very different, vantage points offer anthropologists opportunities to gain a greater understanding of their own cultural biases and how these are often imposed on others.
> (Cornwall and Lindisfarne, 1994, p. 2)

This is a difficult process, which is not always self-affirming. Okely (1992, p. 24) makes the point that, although it may seem 'comfortably neutral for some, this depends on how it is interpreted. In its fullest sense, reflexivity forces us to think through the consequences of our relations with others.' For Callaway (1992, p. 33) it 'becomes a continuous mode of self-analysis and political awareness'. It is this insistence on the 'double frame' (Prell, 1989) of reflexivity which distinguishes nursing and anthropological approaches. For nurses, this entails not only a critical appraisal of oneself, but also challenging assumptions about the cultural construction of our knowledge in order to know and better understand the way in which we construct and practice care.

Nursing rituals

The nursing literature has recently focused on rituals and ritualized practice in nursing (MacLeod and Hockey, 1979; Chapman, 1983; Walsh and Ford, 1989; Walsh, 1990; Hung, 1992; Hatton-Smith, 1994). Rituals in nursing practice are associated with repetitive, mimetic, thoughtless actions and traditions devoid of any empirical basis. Walsh and Ford (1989, p. ix), for example, note that ritual action 'implies carrying out a task *without thinking it through* in a problem-solving, *logical way*'. They point out that nursing practice must be 'a *rational, fact-based* discipline' (Walsh and Ford, 1989, p. 152), abandoning 'ritual and myth and progress to a *rational* research-based footing' (my emphasis). Hatton-Smith (1994, p. 304) defines ritual as 'a task which is carried out without individualized thinking'. When discussing approaches to pre-operative fasting, Hung (1992, p. 287) observes that: 'Attempts are being made to improve the quality of care by a few experienced nurses who refuse to accept these *irrational traditions*' (my emphasis).

From this perspective, nursing rituals are counter-productive to a thinking, rational, logical, scientifically based nursing profession.

The origins of this juxtaposition between ritual and rationality in the nursing literature would seem to lie in Chapman's (1983) study of five hospitals in south London. In this she contrasts Menzies' (1970) psychodynamic model of ritual practices – as defences against stress – with a sociological model which utilizes Bocock's (1974) theory of ritual. I quote this in full from Chapman's article:

> Rational action should not be seen as necessarily irrational or non-rational. Irrational action is action to which certain rational criteria could be applied, and which fails to meet criteria. Some magical action may be of this kind; this type could be replaced by technological action if and when rational criteria were applied. Non-rational action is action which cannot be assessed by any rational criteria because they are inapplicable, for example, the feeling involved in loving a person. Ritual action is best seen as to some extent rational, and also non-rational at times.
>
> (Chapman, 1983, p. 15)

The epistemological implications of this go to the heart of Western philosophical debates concerning 'rational man' – and to anthropological concerns with the ethnocentric, evolutionist implications of attempts to define a universal rationality based on Western presuppositions (Overing, 1985). As Bell (1992) points out, the distinction between technical and ritual action can easily collapse into a distinction between the rational and the irrational. One of the problems with the above statement is the failure to define what is meant by 'rational action'. The same problem afflicts the nursing literature, for what is 'rational' about any nursing action is assumed by the authors to be something we would all know and agree upon. However, as Hobart notes when writing about rationality and reason, rationalists:

> are remarkably loath to define them; and when they do they usually disagree. This is not surprising, as the great champions of reason from Descartes to Leibniz or Kant differed so deeply over what reason was and could do.
>
> (Hobart, 1985, p. 108)

Appealing to rationality 'then becomes a matter of ranking, and certain thought is considered absolutely superior to all others' (Overing, 1985, p. 5). That superior thought is based on Western scientific knowledge.

What is implicit in Walsh and Ford's argument, and in much of the nursing literature on ritual, is the association of an objective rationality with an objective science. Kuhn (1970), Feyerabend (1975) and Rorty (1980), to name but a few, have fiercely criticized this model of scientific rationality. They question the neutrality of science by arguing that the type of understanding being sought 'reflects particular value-laden cognitive interests' (Hobart, 1985, p. 107). While Walsh and Ford (1989, p. x) note that 'there may be a place for intuition in the art of nursing', the emphasis is on the rational, the technical and the scientific. In many ways, this is the obverse of what Schon (1987) proposes that reflection aims to achieve. He notes that technical rationality derives from positivist philosophy:

> Technical rationality holds that practitioners are instrumental problem-solvers who select technical means best suited to particular purposes. Rigorous professional practitioners solve well-informed instrumental problems by applying theory and technique derived from systematic, preferably scientific, knowledge.
>
> (Schon, 1987, p. 3)

He proposes, rather, that practitioners use theories which are generated from their experience, education, values and beliefs. From a different perspective, Benner and Wrubel (1989) also see experience as well as intuition as being central to nursing action and nursing care. Ashurst (1993) has recently criticized the outlawing of various nursing aids, such as the Buxton-type chair and the Sorbo-ring cushion, as a result of critical research. On the basis of his experience, he notes areas where both of these aids improve the care and comfort of patients. Church and Lyne (1994) examined the evidence which has led to the withdrawal of ring cushions in midwifery and, one could add, in many other areas of nursing. Far from conclusively showing that they cause circulatory impairment which predisposes to thrombosis or pressure sores, the research notes only that they are 'believed' to do so or that the patient is 'liable to be affected'. The point is that not only are tentative conclusions elevated to the status of objective 'fact', but also these 'facts' are themselves open to subjective interpretation.

The implications of analysing nursing actions in terms of whether they are rational/irrational/non-rational are not confined to the debate on objectivity, but involve the nature of care itself. Chapman (1983, p. 16) notes that in one hospital in her study, nurses were making up the temperatures, and she suggests that this had 'something to do with an attempt to communicate concern and healing to significant others'. She also points out that doctors and nurses may be observed 'simply touching patients with the apparent intent of signifying care, concern or healing'. For Chapman, these are 'non-rational rituals'. Rather than approaching ritual from this perspective, I want to suggest that ritual can be an important aspect of caring.

Ritual and anthropology

Almost all nursing theorists recognize the importance of religious observance in caring for patients. However, such observances are usually associated with specific practices surrounding death and dying, or else relate to personal hygiene or acceptable diets, such as kosher or halal for Jews and Muslims, respectively. Some theorists also focus on spirituality and the importance of caring for the well-being of the human spirit (Leininger, 1981; Parse, 1981; Watson, 1985; Brykczyńska, 1992). The approach taken here is rather different in that rituals themselves are seen as ways in which individuals care for others. In reflecting on these rituals nurses may better understand how they go about caring for others.

Anthropology has a long history of association with the study of ritual, from Herbert Spencer and James Frazier through to the present day. Given this history, it is perhaps not surprising that anthropologists have proposed numerous theories to explain and understand it. These theories, as Bell (1992) notes, are embedded in broader discourses which reflect the history and dynamics involved in the production of knowledge. It is also not surprising that anthropologists do not always agree about the way in which ritual should be understood (Leach, 1968). Most would agree, though, that ritual is a kind of performance that is not confined to actions associated with religious institutions. For Jean La Fontaine (1972, p. xvii): 'ritual expresses cultural values, it "says" something and therefore has meaning as part of a non-verbal system of communication.'

Gerholm (1988) argues that rituals are not just expressions of abstract ideas, but that they do things and have effects on the world. He also notes that rituals involve work. Bell (1992, p. 123) makes the point that ritual is a practical way of dealing with specific circumstances and is 'never simply or solely a matter of routine, habit, or the "dead weight of tradition"'.

Theories which seek to understand ritual have developed alongside ways in which to describe it. Until recently, anthropologists have largely focused on public rituals, such as those surrounding calendar events or celebrations, or those which concern the alleviation of misfortune. The Belgian sociologist, Arnold Van Gennep (1960), proposed an approach to describe another form of public ritual, namely the 'rites of passage'. These are rituals which accompany the passage of a person or group as they are socially transformed through the life cycle, and they involve a change of place, state, social position or age. They are marked by three phases: separation, marginality (or liminality), and re-incorporation. This approach has been used to describe life-cycle rites, such as birth, puberty, marriage and death, in many societies, and it has also been extended to the secular arena.

More recently, anthropologists have turned their attention to private, domestic or personal rituals (Sered, 1988). This interest has largely developed from an awareness by feminist scholars that public rituals have tended to be associated with 'folk' traditions, or with the 'practical' aspects of religion, rather than with the institutional or transcendental. They have been subsumed as being marginal or subordinate in some way. As Sered (1988) also points out, they are often, but not exclusively, associated with women. Feminist anthropologists have insisted that it cannot be assumed a priori that the domestic and personal rituals which women undertake in order to care for and protect households and families are of less transcendental importance than the public rituals and religious observances which are often dominated by men (Tapper and Tapper, 1987; Sered, 1988). Personal rituals are personalized in that they are concerned with particular, often well-loved individuals with whom one is connected in relationships of care and concern. Sered takes the example of the difference between the Christian theologian's intent in kissing the cross, and that of a woman who kisses the cross in her living room. The woman may be concerned with the life of her sick child, rather than with abstract problems of life and death.

In the following section I shall examine the way in which Gujarati women in east London care for others through ritual. These rituals 'say' something about culturally constructed classifications which inform ideas about the body and person, about relationships with divinity and about gender relations. They are also ways of dealing with particular circumstances in the lives of these women, and of caring for family members. Reflecting on these rituals raises questions which are relevant to nursing care, and which can help us to better understand ourselves and the assumptions we make about our practice.

Personal rituals and care among Gujarati women

The women in this study all performed a variety of personal rituals throughout the Hindu (lunar) year, which are primarily concerned with promoting health and caring for the well-being, good fortune and protection of household members in general, and specific categories of people in particular. Both women and men saw these rituals as being largely the responsibility of women. Ethnographic fieldwork, using participant observation and informal and semi-structured interviews, was carried out in Gujarati households and in four women's groups in east London over a period of 14 months during 1983–1984. The majority of the women in the study came to the UK from the east African states of Tanzania, Kenya, Uganda and Malawi, although some younger respondents came directly from Gujarat, often as brides. Their ages ranged from 18 years to the early 70s, and they came from diverse castes and had a variety of educational backgrounds – from three years' schooling to degree level. The majority did not work outside the home. Gujarati kin relations are hierarchical and patriarchal, and are ideally structured around the patriline – a line traced through men. An examination of their personal rituals also shows the bilateral nature of these relationships within a patrilineal culture where, as married sisters, women care through ritual for their own natal lineage.

The household shrine: daily *puja* (worship) and the care of descendents and ancestors

Unlike Christianity and Islam, Hinduism does not require regular public worship at the temple. Rather, it is the household shrine which is the focus of everyday religious and ritual activity. In other cultures, for example in Taiwan (Stafford, 1992) and Greece (Du Boulay, 1986), household shrines are also an important focus of ritual. The Gujarati household shrine always contains a bell 'to wake the Gods' and a small tray containing a stick of incense and a lamp made from cotton wool and camphor. The deity is embodied in the light of the camphor flame, and its benevolent, protective grace is transmitted to the worshipper and absorbed through the eyes (Fuller, 1992). Food is offered to the deities and the consecrated remains (prasad) are often distributed among the household members in the evening. The essence of worship is *puja*, the 'core ritual of popular theistic Hinduism', when Hindus pay homage to powerful deities whom they honour as revered guests (Fuller, 1992, p. 57). While at the temple, the concerns of the community and larger world may be the focus of concern; in the household, rituals are more often concerned with personal affairs – the health, protection, well-being and good fortune of its members, the resolution of problems, or the ending of suffering or illness.

The household shrine may also contain images or other representations of the lineage deity. This deity refers to a goddess who is specific to a particular patriline, a line traced through males. All Gujaratis, whether born in Gujarat or not, are linked to their ancestral place of origin in Gujarat through their lineage deity, and they have a spiritual relationship with their ancestral place of origin. The deity cares for the prosperity, health and well-being of members of the patriline, and is in turn worshipped and cared for at the household shrine and all major ritual events by the descendents. The deity also informs and authenticates the specific lifestyle or family tradition – the many different rites, customs and conduct – associated with a particular patriline. There are a myriad different practices which distinguish one patriline from another, from the sequence and amount of spices and aromatics used when cooking, to the celebration, or not, of life-cycle rituals.

While men retain their affiliation and identification with their patriline and its deity throughout life, for women the situation is different. As a married woman, it is the religious duty (*dharma*) of a wife to protect the health and longevity of her husband, and one of the ways in which she does this is to perform ritual duties and carry out customs and practices which enhance his welfare and that of his patriline. This means that, with marriage, a woman changes her affiliation, including her lineage deity, from that of her birth household to that of her married household. As one woman said, 'when you get married you take on your husband's *devi*. The devi is an ancestor from way back somewhere.' Another woman observed that, 'when you come to live in your husband's home then there are all these things you have to do that you didn't do in your mother's home.' These 'things' are the traditions and practices associated with the lineage deity. In the case of two sisters, for example, one may undertake the simant ritual in the seventh month of pregnancy, while for the other this may not be the tradition in the patriline into which she marries (McDonald, 1987). Even if the two women do celebrate this ritual, the content may vary according to the tradition of each husband's lineage deity. Men and women thus have different relationships with their lineage deity and experience these rituals in different ways.

Prior to worship, Gujaratis (and other Hindus) must ritually purify themselves by bathing and removing their shoes. Menstruating women cannot worship at the shrine or take part in any ritual activity because their menses render them ritually impure. Similarly, in Islam, menstruating women may not touch the Qur'an, enter the mosque or keep the fast at Ramadan (Delaney, 1991). Traditionally, and even today in many parts of India (Fuller, 1992), menstruating women are separated from other members of the household and excluded from cooking because their relative impurity means that they could pollute others – either through touch or the medium of food, which I shall elaborate on shortly. Among my younger respondents, however, this rule was largely attentuated, although some, while they help to prepare the food, did refrain from cooking. Menstruating women cannot pollute the Gods – humans are unable to do this – but if they participate in rituals they may be held responsible in the future as the cause of misfortune or suffering to themselves or other family members. For Hindus, almost all bodily fluids – such as saliva, faeces, urine, semen and menstrual blood – are potential sources of pollution, as well as hair and nail clippings.

Purity in the ritual sense is not necessarily concerned with bodily cleanliness in the way that this is understood in English. Certain substances in different cultures can have the effect of ritual purification. It is well known that in Hinduism the cow is held to be sacred. Its dung is also used as a purifying agent. In rural India, a birth room may be smeared with cow dung in order to achieve ritual purification from the pollution caused by the mother giving birth. Sacred rituals are performed on ground which has been smeared with cow dung and 'a dying man is lowered on to such a surface' (Hershman, 1977, p. 284). Douglas (1966) suggests that dirt avoidance in European culture is a matter of hygiene and aesthetics and, moreover, that our idea of dirt is dominated by knowledge of pathogenic organisms. Dirt is 'matter out of place', but it is a relative idea. Shoes in themselves are not dirty, but they are considered dirty if placed on the dining-room table; food is not dirty in itself, but it is considered dirty to leave cooking utensils in the bedroom. Our pollution behaviour is the 'reaction which condemns any object or idea likely to confuse or contradict cherished classifications' (Douglas, 1966, p. 36).

Certain aspects of nursing care are also based on a classification process which distinguishes between sterile and non-sterile procedures, tasks and bodily fluids. Some procedures, such as changing a dressing, may require the articles used as well as parts of the nurse (his or her hands) to be sterile. Others, such as giving an injection, are intermediary. The needle is sterile, while the nurse is 'clean'. Non-sterile procedures, such as taking a patient's temperature, require the instrument and the nurse to be 'clean'. This classification process also emphasizes the way in which parts of a ward are categorized as clean or unclean (e.g. the 'pan room'), and tasks as clean or dirty. Similarly, bodily fluids are treated as potentially pathogenic, and capable of contaminating the nurse, who protects himself or herself from these dangers by wearing gloves. Depending on the context, bodily fluids may also be classified as sterile (a midstream urine specimen) or clean (a urine specimen for routine testing), while others are always classified as dirty (faeces). The classification of blood is also context-dependent – it appears to be sterile inside the body but non-sterile outside. However, the potential for contamination from blood also renders it highly dangerous in ways which saliva, for instance, is not, and the rules for dealing with blood and blood products are much more stringent.

Katz (1984) has utilized some of Douglas' (1966) ideas in her discussion of rituals in an operating theatre. She notes that the words 'clean', 'dirty', 'sterile' and 'contaminated' assume different meanings in the theatre and at different stages of the operation. For example, while objects or parts of objects, and people are either sterile or non-sterile, non-sterile objects are further classified as clean, dirty or contaminated. Operations themselves are classified according to the degree of sterility and contamination likely to be present. Eye operations are clean, while colonic operations are dirty. Ritual during most operations is concerned with avoiding contamination of the patient from the outside, but in operations classified as dirty, they are also concerned with contamination of the patient and staff from inside the patient. She also notes that, in the operating room, nurses transform the theatre from being 'dirty' at the completion of an operation to being 'clean' once the walls, floors, furniture and fixtures have been wiped with antiseptic solution. These rituals help to specify categories which can otherwise become confused.

The undertaking of vows (*vrat*)

An important and extremely common way in which Gujaratis care for others through ritual is in the undertaking of vows. While men can and do undertake vows, it is predominantly women who do so in this context. In Western culture, vows are often associated with the Christian tradition, especially in Catholicism, where priests and nuns undertake a vow of chastity and obedience. In some religious orders this also includes a vow of poverty, or even one of silence. In so far as nursing is concerned, Roach (1985) has suggested that commitment is one of five elements of caring behaviour. Brykczyńska (1992, p. 35) points out that a caring commitment 'involves a form of promise or pledge; a professional assurance that the nurse will engage herself in the interests of the patient'.

In Hinduism, a vow is rather like a contractual agreement with the Gods (McGilvray, 1982), which can take many forms. It is a complex ritual which is made up of several components, including the recital of a story from a holy book which details the efficacy of the vow, a period of fasting, and the offering of gifts on its completion (Raheja, 1988; McGee, 1991; Harlan, 1992). The purpose of undertaking vows is to attain the grace of a deity for a specific objective – whether for the care, protection and well-being of the family or specific members by acquiring merit with God, for personal satisfaction and the 'goodness of God' through devotion and discipline, or to achieve a particular wish, often in times of family or personal crisis or during episodes of illness. Here I want to focus on several vows which women undertake in order to care for specific categories of people.

Jaya parvati vrat: the care of husbands

The relationship between husband and wife in Hinduism is often idealized in the relationship betwen Lord Rama and his faithful and obedient wife Sita who followed him into exile. In ancient texts such as the Laws of Manu, the wife is represented as the 'half body' of her husband. He stands in the position of a god to her. One of the ways in which this hierarchical relationship is expressed is that a wife can eat her husband's left-over food which, in other relationships – except those with one's young children – is considered extremely polluting to the recipient. Similar representations of women are found in Islam. Among Turkish women, for example, it 'is considered appropriate for a woman to be totally devoted to her husband, since he is considered a second god and represents God in the world and in the family' (Delaney 1991, p. 33). The Gujarati women in this study were rather dismissive of the idea that their husband was 'some kind of god', as one woman put it, but they did acknowledge that in some areas of their lives they were subordinate to him. Many women in this study were also economically dependent on their husbands. Only one woman had divorced, and for some considerable time afterwards she had been shunned by friends and ostracized from social gatherings. A devoted wife enacts rituals in order to protect and care for her husband throughout life. If she does not do this, he may fall ill or even die, bringing misfortune to the family and tragedy for the wife. A widow was traditionally excluded from rituals and sometimes seen as harbinger of misfortune or the cause of the evil eye. As a widow, a woman removes her marriage bangles, necklace and almost all jewellery, and can no longer place a vermilion mark in her hair parting, all of which symbolize the married state. She wears only white or pale-coloured saris.

Jaya parvati vrat is a ritual performed by women for five years after marriage in order to ensure the health and longevity of their husband, and to protect their own state as an auspicious married woman. It lasts for five days during the lunar month of Asadha (June–July), when women observe a fast which excludes salt, rice and lentils from the diet. Each morning they read from the stories of Parvati – an exemplar of the chaste and loyal wife in the divine world – and worship grain shoots which are grown for the ritual. On the final day of the fifth year, usually armed with a supply of Hindi and Gujarati videos, women observe a vigil throughout the whole of one night and the following day. On that afternoon, five women – or at least an uneven number of women – are invited to the house. These women must, like the wife, be married, not menstruating or pregnant, and with their husband still living. The wife places a red dot on the forehead of each woman, washes the right big toe of each in milk and water and sprinkles it with uncooked rice. The women are given various articles associated with married women – plastic bangles, an auspicious betel nut, a small amount of money, a stainless steel bowl or plate, and perhaps a piece of material for a blouse, and a meal which completes the vow.

Some women continue to perform an annual ritual for one day when they observe a vigil and abstain from salt in the diet in order to protect and nurture the longevity of their husbands. A good and auspicious wife dies before her husband, while a widow is a 'living symbol of inauspiciousness' (Fuller, 1992, p. 23). Among respondents in east London, women from all castes and classes performed this ritual in order to care for their husband after marriage.

Sitala satam: the care of children

Throughout northern India the goddess Sitala is associated with smallpox (Wadley, 1980; Nicholas, 1981), and sometimes measles. While recognizing that smallpox has a physiological cause, it was also believed that, when not properly worshipped, Sitala was the harbinger of the illness. Sitala, or *mataji* (mother goddess), are both terms still used by Gujarati women to describe smallpox, chickenpox and, in some cases, measles. In Gujarat, Sitala is also seen as a protector of children (Wadley, 1980) and it is in this sense, too, that she is worshipped annually at sitala satam. While some younger respondents in east London were concerned not to have children immediately after marriage, none contemplated having no children at all. Hershman (1977, p. 275) notes of women in Hindu society that 'as a mother she has the opportunity to gain status and authority; but as a wife, a woman has very little status at all'. Ideally it is with the birth of sons that a woman is said to fulfil her personhood by providing progeny to continue her husband's patriline, and to perform funeral rites at his death. Ideally, too, sons and their wives care for his parents in old age. Among older female respondents, many were widowed and living in their sons' households. Studies from rural and urban India, however, indicate that there are numerous cases where it is married and unmarried daughters who take on this role.

Sitala satam is a ritual which aims to care for and protect children and promote their good health. It takes place on the seventh day of the dark fortnight in the month of Sravana (July–August), and is preceded by nag panchami (the cobra fifth), when the face of the cobra is worshipped at the household shrine. Women observe a fast on this day, eating mainly cold sweets and especially milk products. On the sixth day (the cooking sixth), large quantities of food are cooked to be eaten cold the following day on sitala satam (sitala's seventh). The story which is told to accompany the vow has many versions, but includes the injunction to leave the hearth unlit, for at midnight the goddess comes to cool herself in the cold ashes.

In theory, the cooker should not be lit on sitala satam, and the cold food prepared from the previous day is eaten. In practice, most women find that they have to heat food and make hot drinks for husbands and children, and so compromise by not eating any heated food themselves. One or two of the gas or electric rings on the cooker are decorated with cotton wool and red powder, and a small tray is placed beside the cooker, containing some betel nuts, green lentils and a ball of millet and ghee – all said to be good omens. A glass of water is also placed on the tray in order to 'cool the goddess'. Sitala is said to come any time after midnight, and according to tradition she rolled in the cool ashes of the hearth. Now, with gas and electric cookers, she comes to check that they are indeed cool, and that her wishes have been carried out. While children remember the ritual for the large quantities of food eaten, they are also taught by their mother the rudiments of the story of Sitala, of the protection she grants them and of her association with illness. For women, this ritual is one of the ways in which they care for their children by seeking divine protection for them.

Failure to worship the deities, or a specific deity, is often given as a reason for illness or perhaps infertility in women. If a woman or one of her loved ones should suffer in such a way, divine assistance is often sought through ritual as a way of alleviating the suffering. This has many resonances with western Christian traditions where recourse is made to prayer, lighting candles in church or at home in front of an image of Jesus or Mary, or kissing a crucifix.

The care of brothers

In northern India, after marriage or on the early death of her father, a woman's brother is often seen as her protector. A brother has a social obligation to care for his sister, and although she has no jural right to maintenance after marriage, a woman is dependent on the goodwill of her brother for protection and perhaps sanctuary in extreme circumstances. A brother can also be appealed to for help and protection in the case of widowhood, especially, for example, if the woman still has young dependent children. Unlike men, women may begin a process of care through ritual for the well-being of their brothers when they are young girls. Logan (1988) describes an annual vow undertaken by Gujarati girls in east London to protect their brothers and/or ensure a good husband. Two other rituals are enacted during the year which formalizes this bond of care throughout adulthood.

Divasni rakhadi is a day in the bright half of the lunar month of Sravana (July–August). Brothers ask their sisters to the evening meal and present them with gifts such as money and/or saris. Sisters send or take with them a *rakhadi* (protective thread) for their brother to wear on their wrist. In east London this thread is often bought from local shops and is made from elastic with a betel nut placed inside a small artificial flower. The betel nut recurs in many rituals and is said to be a good omen that is considered auspicious. Women emphasize the protection and auspiciousness which the rakhadi affords their brother, ensuring his good fortune and health. For a woman, the ritual care of one's brother thus ensures his continuing protection and care. The woman also receives a rakhadi from her brother which ensures her well-being and continuing participation in the rituals of his household.

The second ritual takes place on *bhai bij*, the second day of the Gujarati Hindu New Year. It is perhaps appropriate to note here that the Hindu New Year is celebrated at different times in different parts of India. For Gujaratis, the celebration covers a period of five days. Divali is the last day of the old year. On the second day of the new year the order of visiting is reversed, with brothers visiting their married sisters. The brother's family will usually dine with his sister, and he again gives gifts such as money or saris. Both of these are seen as happy and important ritual celebrations. One man said, 'our sisters are very important to us. We always give to them. We honour them. This is very different from you (meaning me). *Bhai-ben* (brother–sister) for us Gujaratis is very strong.' Bhai-ben can be a relationship of considerable closeness for Gujaratis and others from northern India. Both terms can be used on their own or as suffixes to personal names. A brother or sister may not simply be one's sibling, however, but can include 'cousin brothers and sisters', or all of the men and women from one's village of origin. What it implies is a close relationship but one that excludes sexual intimacy. For a woman, her brother can be a source of help and protection in time of trouble. For a man, his married sister is the most important ritual officiant at all of the life-cycle rites of his children (McDonald, 1993). The gifts given by the brother – the money, clothes and the meal – are also those given to a priest for his ritual services. While women change their patrilineal affiliation at marriage to that of their husband, they continue through ritual to care for the descendents of their natal patriline through their brothers.

Ritual and nursing care

In describing the rituals which Gujarati women enact to care for others, I have sought to contextualize them within the social and cultural setting in which they occur. From this perspective, it is possible to locate these rituals in a wider discourse which links women with care in a subordinate or marginal relationship to androcentric concerns and relations of power. Gilligan (1982), for example, has proposed that women link morality to responsibility and relationships and achieve power and prestige through caring for others. Male development, on the other hand, is linked to justice, fairness, rights and rules. Her theory is critical of the androcentric model of Kohlberg's moral development scale, wherein women's moral judgements seem to remain at the third level of the scale – where morality is equated with helping and caring for others – while men often reach the sixth level, where morality is understood as the subordination of relationship to universal principles of justice.

There have been many criticisms of Gilligan's approach (Larrabee, 1993), not least of which is her failure to address the ways in which women are limited and constrained by their material conditions of existence. One implication of this is that a female caring role has frequently fitted the needs of patriarchal societies. Furthermore, Gilligan fails to take account of the way in which gender is culturally constructed and the many different ways in which it is represented within cultures (Stack, 1993). Stereotyped ideals of masculinity and femininity exist in most cultures, but the way in which individuals experience gender is complex and varied (Cornwall and Lindisfarne, 1994). Linking care to gender, as many male nurses would point out, is difficult to sustain. None the less, her critique, which questions whether relationships and care are subordinate to universal rights, does have implications for nursing. One of the many issues which nursing has had to grapple with is the insistence that the value of care in nursing is no less important than the value of cure in medicine. In the UK today, many nurses are being replaced in management restructuring by people who have little if any connection with the profession. Nurses are being asked to explain what they do by means of check-lists of tasks which can be quantified on computer programs and presented to purchasing authorities who may or may not decide that these tasks require qualified, expert nurses to carry them out. Like the rituals that Gujarati women enact to care for others, much nursing care can seem to be 'invisible' to others. The essence of caring, which nurse theorists and clinicians see as essential to nursing, is again in danger of being subsumed as marginal and subordinate.

Locating these rituals within the kinship structure also invites reflection on the nature of the family and of relationships within it. Membership of the 'extended family', which Gujaratis and other southern Asians subscribe to, is itself situational. Women move at the time of marriage to their husband's household and patriline and, in some circumstances, this family is defined through kin ties with this patriline. In other circumstances, for example, through the enactment of rituals, women are essential members of their own natal patriline and family. Moreover, there is evidence of changing patterns of household composition – to increasingly nuclear households – and allocation of responsibility for the care of elderly members of the family. Difficulties in defining the nature of the family are also apparent in wider society. The fact that kinship relationships are often contextual, flexible and open to negotiation and manipulation has important implications for those individuals, such as health visitors, whose focus of care is primarily on 'the family'.

When we reflect on the rituals themselves, and especially on the ritual complex of vows, several themes emerge which are particularly salient in nursing care. The undertaking of vows includes the recitation of a story, a period of fasting and the offering of gifts on its completion. Gift-giving is commonplace in nursing, but limitations of space preclude more than a passing invitation to reflect on the meaning of these gifts for the donors and recipients, and the nature of the relationships which gifts express. Similarly, another theme which can be isolated in these rituals centres on the creation of auspiciousness. For Gujaratis and other southern Asians, people, objects, events and places as well as planetary influences can be classified as auspicious or inauspicious. Pre-pubescent girls and married women are auspicious in themselves, while widows are often considered to be inauspicious. Objects and substances used in rituals are good omens or portents of future time or events. Periods of time are also seen to be more or less auspicious. Prior to many rituals, an astrologer or a knowledgeable, often older, woman will be consulted with regard to the most auspicious time for the enactment of the ritual. The day is divided into one and a half hour periods which, depending on planetary alignments, are more or less auspicious. If a child is born at an inauspicious time of day, the father may view it through some kind of reflection in order to remove any malign or inauspicious influences from the family. Inauspiciousness can also be related to misfortune and illness, as well as to ideas of pollution or contamination. The rituals which Gujarati women enact aim to care for others by promoting health and well-being and protecting against future illness and misfortune. One of the ways in which they do this is by enhancing auspiciousness and removing inauspicious elements. This invites a reflection on the way in which caring in nursing is also linked with ideas of protection against inauspicious or bad omens and the promotion of auspiciousness – of good portents or signs for future health and well-being.

Fasting

As well as being an important element in the undertaking of vows, women also fast on particular days of the week, lunar month and year. At almost any gathering I have attended, at least one woman, and often more, was fasting. Given the ubiquity with which women fast, it is necessary to understand something of what this entails, both in relation to food itself and in relation to ideas of the body and the person which emerge from this. For nurses, fasting is usually associated with pre-operative 'nil by mouth' requirements to 'starve' the patient. Patients may also be required to be 'nil by mouth' post-operatively although this is not, in my experience, usually referred to as fasting. This idea of the fast is informed by a Judaeo-Christian tradition of total abstention from food or, at least, a fast of 'bread and water'. Fasting entails discipline and may be undertaken as a penance. In lay terms it may be done to 'cleanse' the body of its 'impurities'. In Hinduism, fasting *does not* entail an abstention from food, but rather an avoidance of particular categories of food. There are several distinctions between the food which forms part of the everyday domestic food cycle in northern India and the food of fasts. The latter are 'food of fruits' consisting of uncultivated food, and excluding all cultivated grains and cereals. As Parry (1985) notes, abstention from food is above all abstention from grain and especially rice. Rock salt is substituted for common sea salt, ghee is used instead of oil, and no normal spices or aromatics, except black pepper, are used.

Each day of the week is associated with a particular deity. A woman fasts on the day of the deity in whom she has great faith, either in the hope that a wish will be fulfilled, or to acquire merit through personal service to the deity. Monday is for Lord Siva, Tuesday and Sunday for the Mata (mother goddess), Thursday for a favoured guru who, for many Gujarati women, is Jalarama, Friday is for Santoshima the goddess of contentment, and Saturday is for Lord Hanuman. Wednesday is not usually associated with any deity. Du Boulay (1986) also notes that, in Greece, women keep the saints' days with the saying 'Friday protect your children and Wednesday your husband'. For Christians, and especially Catholics, meat is traditionally excluded from the diet on Friday. For Gujaratis, each day of the week has special rules for the particular deities associated with it. Some fasts are one-meal-a-day fasts, where the fast is continued throughout the day, only those foods associated with the deity being consumed, and the evening meal reverts to the normal domestic food cycle. Other fasts are maintained throughout the day. Fasts are also undertaken at certain times of the Hindu month and year. The eleventh day of the lunar fortnight is an auspicious day when women fast for the entire day. Dried nuts, fruit, yoghurt and potatoes are the mainstays of this fast.

Through the fasts they undertake, women seek the grace and blessings of the deities. For a person to be in a suitable state to receive these, the body and mind-soul must be pure. Fasting, I was told, 'purifies the soul. It shows God you are willing to give up foods for him to get merit from God and a pure soul.' Purifying themselves through the medium of food establishes a spiritual relationship with the deities which enables women to receive grace and blessings from them. The state of blessedness and purity, and the merit acquired from the deities through fasting, empowers women to fulfil a variety of goals, including longevity for their husbands (*jaya parvati vrat*), protection for their children (*sitala satam*), care of their brothers, fecundity, a cure for an illness or alleviation of misfortune and suffering, or auspiciousness of the household. Women have considerable spiritual power (*shakti*), which they use beneficently to care for and protect household and other family members. The enactment of personal rituals empowers women to care for others. They, like women in many other cultures (Du Boulay, 1986; Sered, 1988; Stafford, 1992), are the ritual guardians of the household, who care for the health and well-being of its members.

When we consider what fasting entails for Gujaratis, abstention from rice is of particular importance for them and many other southern Asians. A meal is not considered to be such without rice. Breakfast and lunch, which exclude rice, are referred to as 'snacks' while the food eaten in the evening, where rice forms the 'second course', is regarded as a meal. Rice is the prototypical food. Similar notions exists in Christianity in relation to bread – it is the 'stuff of life' and represents the body of Christ at the Eucharist. Among Turkish Muslims, Delaney (1991) notes that bread is the generic word for food. Where I come from, in rural Australia, a meal was not a meal without the inclusion of meat. In England, there are various terms used to describe 'meal-times', such as breakfast, lunch, tea, dinner and supper, but the meanings of these terms vary from one region to another and between different social classes. Commensality, of course, is more complex than the content of the meal, although it should be noted that the very idea of what is edible is culturally variable. Commensality also includes the range of social relationships involved in eating and the rituals which accompany this. In many cultures, for example, a refusal to share food in a commensal relationship signifies the social termination of that relationship. In many Western cultures, knives, forks and spoons are the common utensils which are used to eat food. Hindus and Muslims do not used utensils in this way, but eat with the right hand. Unlike Muslims, who can share the same bowl or plate, Hindus would consider such sharing highly polluting.

Just what constitutes a meal in terms of content, social relationships and rituals or, indeed, what constitutes food itself, has implications for nursing care. How, for example, is an intravenous infusion of glucose or Hartmans perceived by patients? The fact nurses do not always refer to the patient as 'fasting' when he or she receives intravenous infusions post-operatively may suggest that nurses themselves perceive these as 'food'. The patient is not fasting; he or she is 'nil by mouth'. Parenteral feeding also raises questions as to whether or not patients regard this as food. Ingestion of food normally involves taking it through the mouth and 'eating' or 'swallowing' it. When this process is bypassed by some kind of tubal feeding, what effect does this have on the patient's perception of his or her body?

Differences exist not only in what constitutes food itself and what defines a meal. The way in which food is classified is also culturally variable. The classification of foods as high in protein, carbohydrate, various types of fat, and so on, is itself a Western cultural system of classification which has become part of lay terminology. The food of fasts among Gujarati and other Hindus is also part of an elaborate classification process (Parry, 1985). Fasting, and its association with different days of the week, month and year, has particular relevance for nursing care. Patients with diabetes, for instance, may be undertaking a vow to seek divine assistance from a particular deity in whom they have great faith. As noted earlier, the day or days of the week associated with the deity demand attention to the particular rules of the fast. Patients suffering from renal failure or other illnesses may require a 'special diet'. Such diets themselves often require abstention from biomedical food categories that are deemed to be dangerous, and a positive injunction to eat foods that enhance physical health.

The idea that food is capable of moral transformation, by purifying the mind-soul to receive the grace and blessings of the deities, also involves a rather different idea of the person and the body than that which exists in Western thought. What is central to much Hindu thought and practice in the handling, ingestion and digestion of food is the notion that bodily substance as well as moral disposition are created from food. This is one of the premises on which caste was traditionally based. To ingest food cooked by someone from a lower caste is to take upon oneself the moral qualities of that person. Marriott (1976) has argued that the assumed dichotomy in Western philosophical notions of mind and body is absent from southern Asian Hindu thought. Bodily substance and moral code are two aspects of the same thing. Any transaction, to a greater or lesser extent, involves an exchange of bio-moral qualities which transforms the substance-code of those involved in it. The person in this scheme of things is 'divisible', capable of moral transformation by interaction with others. The body and mind-soul can be morally transformed by the ingestion of certain categories of food. As Parry (1985, p. 628) has stated, in Hindu culture ' a man is what he eats'; his character and temperament are derived from the food that he ingests.

While nursing theory and practice have moved away from the mechanistic medical model of the body and person, this has been replaced by an emphasis on 'holism', in which the nurse cares for the 'whole' unique, individual person (Henderson, 1966; Rogers, 1970; Johnson, 1980; Roy, 1984; Orem, 1985). However, the idea of the individual and of the person varies cross-culturally (La Fontaine, 1986) and within cultures (Moore, 1994). In many Western cultures, personal names are related to individual identity. In Papua New Guinea, Iteanu (1990) has shown that for the Orokaiva, each person can lay claim to an almost infinite variety of such names. Rather than locating separate, personal identities, these names form a system of relations and 'the person who momentarily bears them is simply caught up in it' (Iteanu, 1990, p. 33). La Fontaine (1985) points out that in some cultures personhood is not extended to everyone and, even when it is, it may be a long drawn-out process. Among the Tallensi in Ghana, personhood is only finally validated at death, when divination reveals that the deceased was not simply masquerading as a human being.

The body itself may not be bounded by its outer surface but, through touch, bodily fluids and food are capable of being morally transformed, or of transforming others. Reissland and Burghart (1987), for example, describe the way in which women in Mithila in northern India massage their infants daily in order to instil fearlessness, harden the bone structure, enhance movement and limb co-ordination and increase weight. These practices are based on the idea that between birth and weaning the infant is highly impressionable and its identity can be shaped by the women who massage it. As Savage (1987) observes, the concept of body boundaries is particularly important for nurses because so many procedures – such as injections, enemas, naso-gastric tubes and cervical smears – involve breaching these boundaries. She goes on to note that 'all too often the symbolic meaning these actions may hold for the patient are given scant attention' (Savage, 1987, p. 33).

The identification of AIDS, as well as recent technological discoveries in medical science, have further confounded assumptions that have been made about the body. As Feher has recently observed:

> We must ask ourselves who or what we take the body to be when we perceive it as an immune system threatened on all sides, even by its own function; . . . or when the uterus no longer appears to be the unequivocal, silent locus that perpetuates the species.
>
> (Fehder, 1989, p. 12)

Emily Martin (1992) locates in the language of immunology a body whose external boundaries are wavering while the cells within the body have become invested with agency. She argues that the moral evaluations of these different cells are legitimized by the scientific language of immunology, and reflect societal attitudes towards the morally disordered and undesirable in an era of 'flexible accumulation' in American economic and political life. This idea of the body and bodily disease as a metaphor for society at large has a long history in anthropology (Douglas, 1966) and other disciplines. Sontag (1983), for example, has looked at the way in which cancer – as an uncontrolled, chaotic, malignant growth of cells to be excised and cut out of the body – expresses ideas about undesirable individuals in society, and about unregulated, abnormal, incoherent economic growth in late capitalism in the West. Nurses form part of the wider society and culture in which they live and share in the values and moral dispositions that it represents. However, nurses also care for 'individual' bodies who are often suffering pain and distress. Reflecting on and understanding the metaphorical extensions of the body and bodily illness offers nurses the opportunity to challenge moral evaluations of those whom society regards as morally disordered or undesirable.

Conclusions

From an anthropological perspective, rituals are not about the 'dead weight of tradition' (Bell, 1992), but they express cultural values by saying and doing things and dealing with specific circumstances. Reflecting on the personal rituals which Gujarati women in east London enact provides us with an insight into a different aspect of caring. Personal rituals are particularly relevant to the theory and practice of nursing care because they are situated in everyday life and, as such, say something about our perception of ourselves, our bodies and our relationships with others. This applies not only to those we care for, whether from our 'own' or 'other' cultures, but also to ourselves as nurses. It is not necessary, nor even tenable, to know what these rituals may involve for all the patients we encounter in all their variety and cultural complexity. My purpose has been to stimulate ideas as to how ritual can inform notions of caring. Reflection involves a critical examination of the cultural construction of our own categories and knowledge in order to better understand the assumptions and biases we bring to our encounter with all patients. What anthropology offers is the opportunity to know and better understand ourselves as nurses and the way in which we construct and practise care.

References

Ashurst S (1993) Nurses are wrong to outlaw all ritualistic practices. *British Journal of Nursing* 2, 700.

Atkins S and Murphy K (1993) Reflection: a review of the literature. *Journal of Advanced Nursing* 18, 1188–92.

Bell C (1992) *Ritual Theory, Ritual Practice*. Oxford University Press, Oxford.

Benner P and Wrubel J (1989) *The Primacy of Care*. Addison-Wesley, Menlo Park.

Bocock R (1974) *Ritual in Industrial Society*. Allen & Unwin, London.

Boud D, Keogh R and Walker D (1985) *Reflection: Turning Experience into Learning*. Kogan Page, London.

Brykczyńska G (1992) Caring – a dying art? In Jolley M and Brykczyńska G (eds) *Nursing Care: the challenge to Change*, pp. 1–45. Edward Arnold, London.

Callaway H (1992) Ethnography and experience: gender implications in fieldwork and texts. In Okely J and Calloway H (eds) *Anthropology and Autobiography*, pp. 29–49. Routledge, London.

Caplan P (1988) Engendering knowledge: the politics of ethnography. *Anthropology Today* 4, 8–12.

Carrithers M (1992) *Why Humans Have Cultures*. Oxford University Press, Oxford.

Chapman G (1983) Ritual and rational action in hospital. *Journal of Advanced Nursing* 8, 13–20.

Church S and Lyne P (1994) Research-based practice: some problems illustrated by the discussion of evidence concerning the use of pressure-relieving device in nursing and midwifery. *Journal of Advanced Nursing* 19, 513–16.

Cornwall A and Lindisfarne N (eds) (1994) *Dislocating Masculinity*. Routledge, London.

Coutts-Jarman J (1993) Using reflection and experience in nurse education. *British Journal of Nursing* 2, 77–80.

Delaney C (1991) *The Seed and the Soil*. University of California Press, Berkeley.

Dewey J (1933) *How We Think*. D. C. Heath, Boston.

Douglas M (1966) *Purity and Danger: An Analysis of the Concepts of Pollution and Taboo.* Routledge & Kegan Paul, London.

Du Boulay J (1986) Women – images of their nature and their destiny in rural Greece. In Dubisch J (ed.) *Gender and Power in Rural Greece*, pp. 139–68. Princeton University Press, Princeton.

Feher M (1989) Introduction. In Feher M (ed.) *Fragments for a History of the Human Body. Part One*, pp. 11–17. Zone, New York.

Feyerabend P (1975) *Against Method.* Verso, London.

Fitzgerald M (1994) Theories of reflection for learning. In Palmer A, Burns S and Bulman C (eds) *Reflective Practice in Nursing*, pp. 63–84. Blackwell Science, Oxford.

Fuller CJ (1992) *The Camphor Flame: Popular Hinduism and Society in India.* Princeton University Press, Princeton.

Gerholm T (1988) On ritual: a post-modernist view. *Ethnos* 3–4, 190–203.

Gilligan C (1982) *In a Different Voice.* Harvard University Press, Cambridge.

Harlan L (1992) *Religion and Rajput Women: The Ethic of Protection in Contemporary Narratives.* University of California Press, Berkeley.

Hatton-Smith C (1994) The last bastion of ritualized practice? A review of nursing knowledge of oral health care. *Professional Nurse* 9, 304–8.

Henderson V (1966) *The Nature of Nursing.* Macmillan and Co., New York.

Hershman P (1977) Virgin and mother. In Lewis I (ed.) *Symbols and Sentiments*, pp. 269–92. Academic Press, London.

Hobart M (1985) Anthropos through the looking glass: or how to teach the Balinese to bark. In Overing J (ed.) *Reason and Morality*, pp. 104–34. Tavistock, London.

Hung P (1992) Pre-operative fasting. *British Journal of Nursing* 6, 286–7.

Ingold T (1992) Editorial. *Man (NS)* 27, 693–6.

Iteanu A (1990) The concept of the person and the ritual system: an Orokaiva view. *Man (NS)* 25, 35–53.

Jarvis P (1992) Reflective practice in nursing. *Nurse Education Today* 12, 174–81.

Johnson D (1980) The behavioural systems model for nursing. In Riehl J and Roy C (eds) *Conceptual Models for Nursing Practice*, 2nd edn, pp. 207–16. Appleton-Century-Crofts, New York.

Katz P (1984) Ritual in the operating room. *Ethnology* 2, 335–50.

Kuhn TS (1970) *The Structure of Scientific Revolution.* University of Chicago Press, Chicago.

La Fontaine J (1972) Introduction. In La Fontaine J (ed.) *The Interpretation of Ritual*, pp. ix–xviii. Tavistock, London.

La Fontaine J (1985) Person and individual: some anthropological reflections. In Carrithers M, Collins S and Lukes S (eds) *The Category of the Person*, pp. 123–40. Cambridge University Press, Cambridge.

Larrabee M (ed.) (1993) *An Ethic of Care: Feminist and Inter-Disciplinary Perspectives.* Routledge, London.

Leach E (ed.) (1968) Ritual. In Sills D (ed.) *The International Encyclopedia of the Social Sciences, Vol. 13*, pp. 520–6. Macmillan, New York.

Leininger M (1981) Cross-cultural hypothetical functions of caring and nursing care. In Leininger M (ed.) *Caring: An Essential Human Need. Proceedings of Three National Caring Conferences*, pp. 3–14. Slack, Thorofare, NJ.

Logan P (1988) *The Heart of Hinduism: Domestic Hinduism in Britain.* Seminar paper. Thomas Coram Institute, London.

McDonald M (1987) Rituals of motherhood among Gujarati women in east London. In Burghart R (ed.) *Hinduism in Great Britain*, pp. 50–66. Tavistock, London.

McDonald M (1993) *Caring Women: Gender, Ritual and Power in Gujarati Households in East London*. PhD Thesis, University of London, London

McGee M (1991) Desired fruits: motive and intention in the votive rites of Hindu women. In Leslie J (ed.) *Roles and Rituals for Hindu Women*, pp. 71–88. Pinter Publications, London.

McGilvray D (1982) Sexual power and fertility in Sri Lanka: Battacaloa Tamils and Moors. In MacCormack CP (ed.) *Ethnography of Fertility and Birth*, pp. 25–73. Academic Press, London.

MacLeod CJ and Hockey L (1979) *Research for Nursing*. HM & M Publications, Aylesbury.

Martin E (1992) The end of the body? *American Ethnologist* 19, 121–40.

Marriott McK (1976) Hindu transactions: diversity without dualism. In Kapferer B (ed.) *Transaction and Meaning: Directions in the Anthropology of Exchange and Symbolic Behaviour*, pp. 109–42. Institute for the Study of Human Issues, Philadelphia.

Menzies I (1970) *The Functioning of Social Systems as a Defence Against Anxiety*. Tavistock Pamphlet No. 5. Tavistock Institute, London.

Moore H (1994) *A Passion for Difference*. Polity Press, Cambridge.

Nicholas RW (1981) The goddess Sitala and epidemic smallpox in Bengal. *Journal of Asian Studies* XLI, 21–44.

Okely J (1992) Anthropology and autobiography: participatory experience and embodied knowledge. In Okely J and Calloway H (eds) *Anthropology and Autobiography*, pp. 1–28. Routledge, London.

Orem D (1985) *Nursing: Concepts of Practice*, 3rd edn. McGraw-Hill, New York.

Overing J (1985) Introduction. In Overing J (ed.) *Reason and Morality*. ASA Monograph 24, pp. 1–28. Tavistock, London.

Palmer A, Burns S and Bulman C (eds) (1994) *Reflective Practice in Nursing*. Blackwell Scientific Publications, Oxford.

Parry J (1985) Death and digestion: the symbolism of food and eating in north Indian mortuary rites. *Man (NS)* 20, 612–30.

Parse R (1981) Caring from a human science perspective. In Leininger M (ed.) *Caring: An Essential Human Need. Proceedings from Three National Caring Conferences*, pp. 129–32. Slack, Thorofare, NJ.

Powell J (1989) The reflective practitioner in nursing. *Journal of Advanced Nursing* 14, 824–32.

Prell R-E (1989) The double frame of life history in the work of Barbara Myerhoff. In Personal Narratives Group (eds) *Interpreting Women's Lives*, pp. 241–58. University of Indiana Press, Bloomington.

Raheja GG (1988) *The Poison in the Gift: Ritual, Prestation, and the Dominant Caste in a North Indian Village*. University of Chicago Press, Chicago.

Reissland N and Burghart R (1987) The role of massage in south Asian child health and development. *Social Science and Medicine* 25, 231–9.

Roach SM (1985) A Foundation for Nursing Ethics. In Carmi A and Schneider S (eds) *Nursing Law and Ethics*, pp. 170–7. Springer–Verlag, Berlin.

Rogers M (1970) *The Theoretical Basis of Nursing*. FA Davis, Philadelphia.

Rorty R (1980) *Philosophy and the Mirror of Nature*. Basil Blackwell, Oxford.

Roy C (1984) *Nursing: An Adaptation Model*, 2nd edn. Prentice Hall, Englewood Cliffs, NJ.

Salvage J (1985) *The Politics of Nursing.* Heinemann, London.

Savage J (1987) *Nurses, Gender and Sexuality.* Heinemann Nursing, London.

Scholte B (1972) Toward a reflexive and critical anthropology. In Hymes D (ed.) *Reinventing Anthropology,* pp. 430–52. Pantheon Books, New York.

Schon D (1983) *The Reflective Practitioner.* Temple Smith, London.

Schon D (1987) *Educating the Reflective Practitioner.* Jossey-Bass Publishers, San Francisco.

Sered S (1988) The domestication of religion: the spiritual guardianship of elderly Jewish women. *Man (NS)* 23, 506–21.

Sontag S (1983) *Illness as Metaphor.* Penguin, Harmondsworth.

Stack C (1993) The culture of gender: women and men of color. In Larrabee MJ (ed.) *An Ethic of Care,* pp. 108–11. Routledge, London.

Stafford C (1992) Good sons and virtuous mothers: kinship and Chinese nationalism in Taiwan. *Man (NS)* 27, 363–78.

Street A (1992) *Inside Nursing: A Critical Ethnography of Clinical Nursing Practice.* State University of New York Press, Albany.

Tapper N and Tapper R (1987) The birth of the prophet: ritual and gender in Turkish Islam. *Man (NS)* 22, 69–92.

Van Gennep A (1960) *The Rites of Passage.* Routledge and Kegan Paul, London.

Wadley SS (1980) Sitala: the cool one. *Asian Folklore Studies* 39, 33–62.

Walsh M (1990) From model to care plan. In Salvage J and Kershaw B (eds) *Models for Nursing* 2, pp. 39–45. Heinemann, Oxford.

Walsh M and Ford P (eds) (1989) *Nursing Rituals: Research and Rational Action.* Butterworth-Heinemann Ltd, Oxford.

Watson J (1985) *Nursing: the Philosophy and Science of Caring.* Colorado Associated University Press, Boulder.

Further reading

Carrithers M (1992) *Why Humans Have Cultures.* Oxford University Press, Oxford.

Sered S (1988) The domestication of religion: the spiritual guardianship of elderly Jewish women. *Man (NS)* 23, 506–21.

8

The emotional cost of caring

Verena Tschudin

Caring compassion can drain us emotionally, and the psychological cost of caring can result in professional burn-out and/or disillusionment. It is not easy to maintain the balance between professional integrity, concepts of duty, personal preferences and ever increasing structural demands on time and energy. Caring can be an emotionally one-way process; instead of energizing us, it can deplete our inner resources until we become spiritually bankrupt.' This chapter looks at how this phenomenon comes about, and what can be done to avoid such a negative consequence of caring. Counselling can interrupt this downward trend of maladaptive caring behaviours but, most significantly, we need to talk more openly about the emotional cost of caring and build into our notions of care concern for the carer – a deliberate and wise concern for the mental and spiritual nature of the carer.

Introduction

The 'Three Es' driving the health service – economy, effectiveness and efficiency – undermine knowledge, care and understanding. This was the message Christine Hancock, General Secretary of the Royal College of Nursing, gave to a Conference of the National Association for Staff Support (NASS) on 4 May 1994.

This is a simple analysis of a complex situation, but perhaps it has to be put simply for it to be realized. Hancock might have said that the 'three Es' are in opposition to reflective practice as the essence of caring. The ideologies of the market-place and of caring do not mix well. In other words, 'the system' destroys care.

Those who care often feel that they do so against almost impossible odds. They constantly swim against the tide.

It is not surprising that nurses have seen their advocacy role as an increasingly important element with which to fight 'the system'. Nurses want to maintain their ideal of caring and seek for more or better ways to defend this. Some of these ways are heroic or altruistic, and inevitably this can lead to disappointment and failure, reinforcing the problem that 'the system' is to blame. A vicious circle is thus created from which there is no escape.

'The problem' of the emotional cost of caring is complex, as will be discussed in this chapter.

The emotional need

Nursing is still seen as giving a high level of job satisfaction. At the same time, myths and images persist of nurses being born rather than made. 'Holding, talking and preparing a cup of tea' come to a nurse naturally and 'effortlessly, with little demand on herself and for little material reward' (Smith, 1992, p. 4). The public rarely sees and appreciates the other tasks of nurses: cleaning incontinent patients; dressing wounds which are painful, smelly and infectious; the unsocial hours; being blamed by angry and tense patients and colleagues; being injured by patients and equipment – or the lack of it; having to break bad news; and trying to balance a budget against the most incredible odds. These issues are a million miles from 'holding, talking and preparing a cup of tea'. Still, however, nurses go on working against all these odds, wanting to continue with nursing. Why?

The word nurse has French and Latin roots of 'nourishing', that is, people who are nurses nourish others. A simple look at the symbolic image of the nourisher brings an element into view which is perhaps not often recognized. Symbols function mainly in and from the unconscious and in pictures rather than in clear concepts (Chetwynd, 1982).

The archetype of the nurse, like all archetypes, is complex and can be confusing. Archetypes are 'conscious representations' or 'primordial images' or 'motifs' which 'can vary a great deal in detail without losing their basic pattern'. 'They are without known origin; and they reproduce themselves in any time or in any part of the world' (Jung, 1964, p. 58). The archetype of the nurse is that of healer and nourisher. This image can be very powerfully connected with an actual nurse when someone is ill and the nurse provides the necessary 'nourishment' in the form of care and support. A very strong bond can be created between the sick person and the nurse, helping the patient or client through a difficult phase or experience.

The negative image or shadow of the archetype is the keeper of sickness and refuser of comfort, support and health. Every archetype has a positive and negative (or shadow) image. Confusion can arise when a sick person looks for a 'nurse' or some such person to supply his or her needs. When a nurse cannot or does not supply these needs, an already sick person can become very ill. Because this is an unconscious need and something archetypal rather than clearly perceived, the acknowledgement of the need is very difficult to access, either for the sick person or for someone who might indeed be able to help.

The inner, unconscious and symbolic life is not easy to understand or to come to terms with. Sooner or later, however, most people either gain glimpses of it or are powerfully confronted with it. It is then that we become aware that outer and inner lives must balance, and the need to look inwards becomes imperative. Inevitably this is different for every person, but needs for security, help and nourishment are very common – particularly when someone is ill. It is then that the inner nurse comes into focus in the form of a need – indeed a craving – to be 'nursed', 'mothered', or 'nourished' physically, emotionally, or spiritually. When this has been understood by a person, he or she may begin to realize, often painfully, that such a figure does not exist, or does not exist any more in reality. The memory of a nanny or children's nurse may have given rise to the present image. Now, however, the person himself or herself has to function as nurse to the self. Drawing on the symbol, that person may need to learn to become truly adult, stand on his or her own feet and supply his or her own needs. Thus the symbol of the nurse can then function from the positive aspect, that is, helping the person to undertake this nursing of the self.

Nurses must be nurses to themselves first of all before they can really be nurses to others, in the same way that mothers must be mothers to themselves before they can really be mothers to their children, doctors must be doctors to themselves, priests must be priests to themselves, and so on.

This is not something which can be taught in a class. It is not even something which happens in the first few years of being a nurse; rather it dawns, perhaps gradually, perhaps with a jolt, but mostly by one's own efforts and not because one is told about it. Those people who are aware of it use this insight with caution and precision; those who are not aware of it can nevertheless also use it, but it has then quite a different power. However, those who imitate it stand out like sore thumbs as the 'do-gooders' whose own unfulfilled needs get in the way of any true care.

Many young people embark on a nursing career because of a deep and unconscious need to be nourished and cared for. They seek the fulfilment of this need through their own caring, and their work is a cry for fulfilment of their own inner person. The fact that many nurses go on working against all odds and every obstacle shows that this need to be cared for is immense and all-pervasive.

It would be incorrect to say that this means that only very needy people go into nursing. There are a great many very needy people in all the helping professions. This does not demean the helping and caring professions – perhaps they exist for the practitioners more than for their clients anyway – but it gives them a different dimension. Since we are all damaged and needy in some way, perhaps this creates that bond which is often so strong among 'sets' of nurses, wards and departments and gives nurses a strong sense of possessiveness of patients and territory.

Any emotional need goes very deep. For nurses it is the acknowledged and unacknowledged need to be a person, to be taken for someone important, to be seen to be doing something good and to be able to say, at the end of the day, that the world is a better place because of what was done. These things constitute the real need. They are connected with the positive side of the symbol of the nurse. When these needs are not fulfilled, then there arises the need to control and rule, so as not to be at the mercy of someone or something else. The shadow of the symbol, the controller and guardian of negative influences and of ill health, then predominates.

The needs to be acknowledged as a person are deep and real, and are often confusing and get in the way of caring. When they are understood and given a name they are no longer threatening, but become tools for working with and achieving great things. However, if unacknowledged they can deteriorate and wreak havoc.

Clearly, these types of needs are not easily met by an institution the aim of which is to balance the books. Simply giving nurses more money does not solve the problem. Because the needs cannot be met easily does not mean that they go away; they simply get distorted. The outcome is a perpetual anger against 'the system' and abnormal behaviour of the workers, including emotional detachment, disturbances and professional distancing, black humour, smoking and alcoholism. Apparently there may be as many as 40 000 alcoholic nurses in the US (National Association for Staff Support, 1992b).

This, then, is the need which we are addressing, but because it is mostly a hidden and unconscious need, it is not easily addressed. The factors which can be addressed, because they are seen, are the emotions. These are the key to an understanding of what is happening.

The emotional cost

One part of the emotional cost of nursing can be measured in terms of medical conditions (hypertension, cardiovascular disease, depression, etc.) and in terms of absenteeism and days lost through sickness by the institution. However, to the individual this is only part of the story. The individual nurse or health-care worker knows that there are powerful emotions at work characterized by anger, guilt, shame, impotence, helplessness and humiliation.

The culture in which nursing functions is so powerful that even without a word being said, nurses learn what is acceptable and what is not. The idea of nursing as a 'vocation' is coming back into vogue with the National Vocational Qualification (NVQ) (Kershaw, 1994), and it remains to be seen whether this means that 'vocation' will again have the same emphasis of selfless and obedient work for long hours and little pay. If this is not at the moment in any contract, the culture still implies that nurses will conform to the image. The image of the nurse as 'holding, talking and preparing cups of tea' (Smith, 1992, p. 4) fits the archetypal nourishing nurse; it does not fit the shadow archetype of the nurse who cannot or will not heal and who prolongs suffering by following the demands of 'the system'. The dichotomy between the various demands is quite sufficient to render any nurse angry, frustrated, helpless and damaged.

Anger is often the most obvious and destructive emotion, and is therefore feared by both the perpetrators and the recipients. The 'angry person's sense of grievance is ultimately generated not by the situation itself, but by how he or she sees the situation' (Parry, 1990, p. 26). This means that often there is no objectivity and no real relationship to the facts. It is impossible to argue differently with an angry person. An angry person does not want to stop feeling angry, or to be mollified. He or she simply wants to be justified, and will therefore bend views and facts until they seem to give further cause for anger.

All feelings are irrational in the sense that they cannot be rationally explained, but this does not make them any less real. On the contrary, because feelings exist they have to be taken seriously. Other people will not feel the same, even in the same circumstances. Since feelings are based on memories and experiences which are unique to a particular person, they have to be dealt with in a way which is unique to the individual.

Anger, in the way that a nurse might experience it as a result of emotional work, can be destructive to the self and to others. Some of the antisocial behaviour and speech indulged in by some nurses is only one means of trying to deal with the problem. The situation is rather like constantly eating bad or indigestible food, which accumulates in the stomach and at a certain moment is 'vomited' back up, causing pain and confusion to those who do not know what has happened. When anger is acknowledged it can be transformed from being a destructive element to a helpful source of energy. The positive archetypal image can surface again and become active and care for the inner need of the person.

Guilt is a complex emotion. Parry has described it as 'a feeling of moral responsibility for some bad action which hurts or damages another' (Parry, 1990, p. 28). Dryden (1994) describes two different aspects of guilt: one which is 'an unconstructive emotion' and one which is 'constructive remorse'. He further describes 'episodic guilt', that is, guilt rooted in particular episodes when a moral code or ethical principle has been broken, or when the focus is on the consequences of what was done or not done. There is also 'existential guilt', which is linked to a particular dogmatic attitude towards oneself. 'This type of emotion is enduring and is not necessarily limited to particular episodes' (p. 2), and it is characterized by 'four dogmatic attitudes: demandingness, awfulizing, low frustration tolerance and self-blame' (p. 4).

Constructive remorse can be very helpful because it leads to insight and understanding, and the person is probably able to take responsibility by atoning for the bad act in some way which then provides a feeling of forgiveness.

Unconstructive emotion is a feeling of having done wrong when there was no real wrong to be done. It is a feeling of self-punishment which is a kind of indulgence and sometimes a shield from wanting or having to take responsibility for an action. It is an 'existential guilt', which can also mean that one takes on too much responsibility: 'everything that happens to go wrong is my fault'. The 'guilty' person lives by a moral code which admits no wrong and tolerates no deviations, but these wrongs and deviations are far in excess of practical reality; therefore their punishment is a sense of always failing and always having to be punished. This punishment is neither necessary nor administered by someone; it is entirely self-chosen and self-perpetuated. However, this is often not easily seen or acknowledged, hence the severe damage which can be caused by this emotion. Dryden (1994) shows that people can be helped by differentiating between guilt and constructive remorse. Once this has been realized, there is every chance of seeing a situation in its right perspective, and guilt then ceases to be destructive.

It sometimes seems as if nursing and nurses are governed by guilt. If and when nurses can make the distinction between guilt and constructive remorse, then they might be on the way to solving many of their inherent problems.

Shame is the sense of wanting to hide or disappear. It is produced by a feeling of being watched, judged and found wanting – someone or something has found us out. As with anger, which we believe to be generated by others, shame is in fact self-generated – we are our own judge. Until this insight can be reached, however, a lot of unravelling and being listened to is required. Shame often follows on from guilt, and when the latter guilt is understood as basically unnecessary, shame is no longer an issue. When constructive remorse has been recognized as a consequence of having done something wrong, it calls for support and forgiveness, and shame also loses its grip.

Impotence is a feeling of knocking and knocking on a door, knowing that a person is inside, but never getting an answer, or never being taken seriously, and being denied one's human rights. It is a feeling of constantly being belittled and ridiculed. Perhaps this does not happen deliberately, but this is how it is understood by the person concerned.

Depending on temperament and character type, one person may experience impotence in a situation, while another can shrug it off or deal with it in a witty or a rude way. However, for the person who experiences impotence, it is no help to be told to be assertive; this would only be reinforcing the impossibility of the situation. In order to help such a person, one must listen to what has gone into the understanding of the impotence felt, and perhaps help the person to see what might take its place if it were removed.

Humiliation is often the outcome of a feeling of impotence. It is a sense of being exposed in front of others, and of feeling bad, worthless and guilty.

Unlike the other feelings, this emotion is not without foundation. People can treat each other in shocking ways in order to get what they want. A feeling of humiliation may therefore deliberately be placed upon someone for another's personal gain. When someone is taken as a means to another's end, humiliation can result – and is perhaps intended to be the result.

For the person concerned this is a shocking way of being treated groundlessly. For someone who tries, through caring, to be encouraging, helping and caring, to be humiliated is doubly painful.

Yet this is something which happens all the time. Managers and leaders are no stronger or more secure as people than anyone else, and suffer from the same unconscious problems of needing to live out an archetype and probably meeting its shadow rather than the positive image. In an effort to stay afloat, inhuman behaviour to others is not uncommon. What is also not uncommon is a splitting of personal and professional ways of behaving, in sometimes drastic ways, in order to reduce the problem. Nurses tend to deal with such feelings in unhealthy ways because they are unable or unsure how to achieve this in alternative ways. These methods have been well described by Barber (1993) and are considered here under his headings.

Depersonalization occurs when patients are referred to by their medical condition. Patients become not only a diagnosis but also something to be managed by diagnosis rather than as a person.

Detachment and a denial of feelings is expected of staff. 'Getting involved' is discouraged, as is any show of emotion. To reinforce this, staff are disciplined rather than helped to cope in difficult situations.

Reduced decision-making occurs when ritual and routine are adhered to and fostered as a way of coping with workload and feelings.

Responsibility is diluted and individual action is discouraged by overzealous recording. This leads to mistrust of people and their skills, and fear of failure is a constant motivator.

Collusive redistribution of responsibility takes part. 'Authoritative parts of oneself are displaced on to seniors and irresponsible parts on to juniors; consequently seniors are seen as parents and juniors as "childlike". Personal power is denied and professional autonomy and personal initiative are largely left unused.'

Avoidance of responsibility occurs because roles are obscured and boundaries are blurred and undefined. There is scope for excuses, and conflict is ignored.

Delegation of responsibilities then becomes routine. It is easier to 'pass the buck' than to deal with a problem oneself. The higher up a person is in a hierarchy, the more unclear are the responsibilities and the easier it is to blame his or her superiors for inaction.

Idealization of a position occurs. 'Maturity and responsibility are allocated to rank rather than to individual merit.'

Avoidance of change results. This means that no practical change can take place in a ward or area, and also that people cannot change because they are locked into systems of behaviour and belief which function as defences rather than allowing for creativity and growth.

Such basically destructive behaviours are all too common. They function as defence systems and are often inculcated into junior staff at a very early stage. This gives the juniors an even wider sense of the gap between theory and practice, because they are not able to judge accurately what is defence and what is helpful practice. This may be the crucial moment when the positive and negative images of the symbol of the nurse get confused.

The shadow of the symbol is not simply negative. It tends to be seen as negative because it is not well recognized and therefore rejected. In its negative aspect it is destructive, but when seen as shadow and necessary to full integration, these aspects can also be used in the search for a fuller understanding of a particular person or, as here, of nursing and its needs.

The material cost

In *The Costs of Stress and the Costs and Benefits of Stress Management* (1992b), NASS has documented the high cost of stress and bad management of stress. These costs are seen from the viewpoint of individual and organizational health, but also from the financial angle. They make fascinating – and depressing – reading. To quote just two figures: 'Sickness and absenteeism alone costs business approximately £5 billion per year' and 'Around 30 million days are lost at work for certified psycho-neurotic disorders. The cost equals £4 billion a year and excludes psychosomatic complaints and uncertified absence.' The statistics and figures quoted here relate to stress and its consequences, but do not stipulate the causes of stress.

Wheeler and Riding (1994) studied occupational stress in general nurses and midwives, and found the sources of stress to be fourfold:

- work overload and time pressure;
- organizational and management issues;
- poor relationships;
- poor working conditions and facilities.

Wheeler and Riding quote studies in the USA which stipulate that 'workload and relationship problems were important factorial sources of nurse stress'. A general conclusion of their study is that staff nurses experience relatively more stress than other nurses, and they explain this in terms of frustration at not being able to make autonomous decisions and have them carried out.

Owen, in a literature review of stress, coping mechanisms and support systems, found that stress could be classified as 'intrapersonal, concerning forces arising from within the individual; interpersonal, or forces occurring between individuals; and extrapersonal, meaning forces occurring outside the individual' (Owen, 1993, p.8).

These elements point to the fact that stress is a complex issue which, however, is increasingly well understood, taken seriously and analysed in terms of cost. So far it seems that this cost has not been considered too high either for individuals or for industry and society, as only a few positive steps have been taken to reduce stress and therefore costs. There are, however, apparently moves under way to put stress at work on an equal footing with health and safety.

The rest of this chapter will consider some of the supports that are necessary for implementing such ideas and are in some cases already available to health-care professionals.

Types of support

Caring for other people is costly in emotional as well as material terms. Those who care should be supported, regardless of the reasons for stress, and when the reasons are known they should be addressed. The concern of this chapter is the emotional support of carers, but this can only be seen in the context of many other types and systems of support, and they are mentioned here only in outline.

Education and training will always need to be high on the list of any programme of support. This will need to include practical skills of nursing and caring in the area of specialty of the nurse. Updating to learn new techniques and procedures are essential. This should also include professional education and study days in actual and related areas of interest and concern to the individual. Some of these elements will be compulsory under PREP (United Kingdom Central Council for Nursing, Midwifery and Health Visiting, 1995), but this does not mean that employers should therefore be able to abdicate responsibility for educating their staff. Knowledge and understanding of stress and its implications should also come under this heading, because recognizing the signs and symptoms of stress in oneself and others can lead to a reduction in the severity of those symptoms.

Management of stress is vitally important. There are countless possible and advertised methods of stress management. Some of these are more suitable for a particular person or situation than others, and some are more effective than others, but no possibility should be discounted without some trial or recognition. Techniques for the management of stress range from meditation to jogging, and from massage to psychoanalysis.

How a person manages stress is an individual matter. People are frequently unaware of the diverse ways and means of stress management, and therefore they do not have access to the method that would be best for them. As well as sending staff to educational study days and sessions, seminars on stress management should be made available by employers. They may be fostering staff welfare just as much in this way as by more traditional means of education and training.

Management of stress can be both individual and corporate. Some people prefer to sit alone in silent meditation for a while and in this way let the strains of the day drain out of the body. Others prefer group discussions. Sometimes a problem is better dealt with in an individual way, while at other times it is better to consider it along with others.

The important element in any strategy for stress management is firstly the recognition of stress and strain and secondly finding and knowing the most creative way of dealing with it. This has to be learned and practised; it is not simply a matter of 'should know' or of common sense.

Staff support is something which is often acknowledged with lip service rather than deeds. No one would deny that support for staff is a good thing – but that is often the extent of the commitment. If staff support is to be established in a hospital or community, then it cannot be left to management alone. Everyone who is concerned to receive support, in whatever way, has a duty and a responsibility to seek and create the support necessary. The *Charter for Staff Support* (National Association for Staff Support, 1992a) (see Appendix) gives a clear outline of what can and should be done from the point of view of staff and management.

Specific support for staff will include both personal and corporate help, support and counselling. This may mean the possibility of a debriefing after a traumatic event for a nurse, or a long-term commitment to have a member of staff receive counselling. Enlightened employers see this as an investment in a valued member of staff. Christine Hancock, General Secretary of the Royal College of Nursing (RCN), cited the case (at the conference mentioned above) of an employee of the RCN who was receiving long-term counselling after a bereavement and saw this as benefiting both the employee and the employer.

Staff support can be any formal and informal system which is concerned with the mental welfare of the individuals. Much informal support takes place in cafeterias and staff changing rooms. More formal support can be provided in weekly unit or ward meetings. Sometimes this has to be spelled out as 'support', sometimes not, depending on the people and circumstances involved.

When implementing staff support it is important to be as flexible as possible, and to consider in the first instance the person rather than any structures. If support groups or systems become inflexible, then they can do more damage than good. Since the help which they should provide is there to manage change of one kind or another, support systems should normally be concerned with the processes of the individuals, rather than with their own structures.

A great deal has been written about staff support (Owen, 1993) from many different angles and viewpoints, reflecting the many differing needs and situations that arise. In general, it can be said that if there is a practical need, then practical help should be given, and if there is an emotional need, then emotional help should be available. In many situations there is initially a practical need, and an emotional need develops later. People who are skilled in helping will recognize the difference and gear their help appropriately. The different ways in which this can be done will now be explored in more depth.

Emotional support

The aim of any form of emotional support must surely be that the person concerned can function well and appropriately. This must be seen in terms of the Kantian imperative that every person should be treated as an end and not as a means. Quite clearly, however, an employer in health care is concerned that patients receive optimum care, and therefore a fully functioning employee is also the means to that end. Yet the *Charter for Staff Support* (National Association for Staff Support, 1992a) states as its first principle that 'staff in health care services have individual rights to be valued and respected just as any other citizens have', and therefore this must be the basis on which support is given and demanded.

When staff are supported, they are much less likely to show some of the inappropriate behaviours outlined above. Indeed, a study among hospice nurses showed clearly that 'those nurses who felt that their direct supervisor was available to support them used fewer "blocking tactics" with patients' (Nursing Standard, 1994). Various approaches can be used to help another person, depending on the situation, the need and the skills of the helper (and to some extent the client). Some of these approaches will now be outlined.

Crisis intervention is typically used in emergencies or during challenging or hazardous events. The 'objective of . . . crisis intervention is the restoration of psychological balance to at least what it was prior to the crisis' (Stewart, 1992, p. 59).

Stewart (1992) mentions as the first type of crisis intervention 'appropriate social and material assistance'. It depends entirely on the circumstances of the crisis – a major accident, a bereavement, an outburst of anger – what this assistance might be. It could be a cup of tea and sharing memories of a loved person, sitting together in silence, crying and holding each other, attentive listening, giving necessary information, or helping to fill in forms.

The venting of feelings is often considered to be socially unacceptable; therefore a helper who can allow this to happen is doing important work. At other times it may mean helping a person to express feelings which are too deep even to be felt as such; the person may simply be aware of emotional pain.

In a crisis, neither the expression nor the suppression of feelings should be forced. What matters is that the person has the attention of someone with a non-judgemental attitude, so that the essence of the crisis can be brought to the surface. By adopting this stance it is easier to see that an angry person, for instance, is not necessarily angry with the helper, even though his or her verbal and non-verbal language may indicate this. Someone who is angry needs another person to whom that anger can be expressed; a brick wall will not do. However, trying to argue with an angry person, or telling him or her that *you* are really the one who should be angry will not do either. Bringing in other elements simply distorts and inflates such a crisis. Only when the heat of the crisis is reduced can any reasoning or arguing take place. Similarly, in crises such as bereavements or other situations of loss, there should first be free expression of what needs to be said or done. The person should then be assured that in abnormal situations abnormal behaviour is in fact normal. When the immediate shock of the crisis has worn off, then there should be a more positive focus. This may involve some quite specific suggestion such as making an important telephone call, focusing on a positive aspect which might have been mentioned, or an assurance that tomorrow will be a new day. This is a very important aspect of helping in a crisis, as it helps to 'earth' the crisis and the person, and gets the situation back into focus and reality. An offer of further help should always be made, as this is another reassurance to the person that he or she is valued and taken seriously.

The aim of any crisis intervention is to help the person to reach an awareness of his or her feelings about the problem and the ability to express them, to gain a perception of the problem and also to be able to ask appropriately for help by developing personal skills (Jones, 1990).

Long-term counselling would normally follow on the work done during or just after a crisis. This is the emotional work done to integrate insights and experiences, to make sense of them and to move forward and change as necessary. Unless there is some anchoring of insights and experiences, they lose their significance and can leave the person damaged rather than moving forward. This can be the case particularly in experiences of loss such as bereavement, injury, failure of relationships, and perhaps job moves which proved to be disastrous.

The precise meaning of 'long-term' is relative and depends on the situation of the client. After an acute crisis, it may be necessary to meet several times over a period of a few days with a trained worker or in support groups. After a significant loss it may be more necessary to meet regularly, perhaps weekly, for a month or two, using some form of psychological therapy.

Some people find that optimum individual support is a counselling relationship which is ongoing, sometimes for months, but only involves meeting once a month. In such a setting deep issues of the personality can be examined and changed if necessary.

One particular element of such long-term work is a contract. 'Only when both the user and the recipient explicitly agree to enter into a counselling relationship does it become "counselling" rather than the use of "counselling skills".' (British Association for Counselling, 1990). What the contract is or means depends on both parties agreeing to some framework. The contract may be verbal or written, but will necessarily stipulate the length of each meeting, the number of meetings, and any cost or other agreed elements involved.

With this type of help, the skills and methods of the counsellor, therapist or helper are pivotal. Anyone wanting to practise as a counsellor or therapist will need some recognized training and qualification which must be able to be checked. Such people may work in particular modes, that is, they may use Gestalt therapy, neuro-linguistic programming, transactional analysis, psychosynthesis, or any other process. Before entering into such a relationship it may be useful to be clear what these approaches entail and how they are being used. Many counsellors prefer not to be tied to a particular school or approach, but to be eclectic and use whatever method is most appropriate for the client or the particular situation brought to individual meetings.

The effectiveness of counselling does necessarily also depend on the client and his or her willingness to work. A counsellor is not a 'Mr/Ms Fix-It', but rather an enabler or midwife. However, at the outset a counsellor may have to help a client quite considerably to tell his or her story by the use of counselling skills.

The aim of this kind of counselling is 'to provide an opportunity for the client to work towards living in a more satisfying and resourceful way' (British Association for Counselling, 1990). Essentially, counselling is there to help others to help themselves in the emotional spheres of their lives. This does not mean that people should be trained to be totally self-sufficient, but rather that they can be and behave more effectively, resourcefully and satisfyingly.

Owen quotes from a study by Wood (1990) which 'attempts to evaluate methods of psychotherapy, comparing a problem-solving approach with counselling for occupational health nurses', and finding that the problem-solving approach was more successful 'when judged by outcomes over a period of time' (Owen, 1993, p. 14). It must surely depend on what is actually implied by these terms. Egan (1994, p. 12) advocates a systematic and flexible, humanistic, broadly based problem-management and opportunity-development model or framework. The only difference is that Wood speaks of a 'problem-solving' approach and Egan of a 'problem-management' model. Nurses and health-care personnel generally tend to think in terms of problems to be solved by their interventions, whereas all too often in life problems cannot be solved but can be managed with different attitudes and mindsets. It is difficult to be dogmatic here, and all that can perhaps usefully be said is that the approach depends on the people and the circumstances. However, problem-solving (or managing) and counselling are not mutually exclusive.

Problem-management approaches, like those of Egan (1994), Carkhuff (1987), Nelson-Jones (1993) and Tschudin (1995), to mention but a few of the many available, use a systematic model for helping. Such models must be clear, widely applicable and also flexible. What all the authors of such models say is that they are *models* and not 'musts', and servants, not masters. The client should never suffer because a model is followed too strictly or rigidly. When a helper is skilled, models and frameworks may no longer play any significant role because helping is then almost second nature and invariably done in the 'right' way anyway.

All models start with a basic setting of the scene – the 'story' has to be told. This is usually the longest part of the process, because from the story has to be gathered what the real problem is – which is often not the same as the one presented. A useful question here is 'what is happening?'

As the story unfolds, emphasis has to be placed on the feeling involved. Even when anger or some other strong feeling is an early focal point, this may only be a decoy for other significant feelings and meanings. There is therefore a search for a purpose: 'what is the meaning of it?'

Once a central core has been seen or found, this must be captured and transformed into something active. Egan (1994) says that this is the core of counselling, because it is often difficult to carry insights into practice. The question now might be: 'what is your goal?' or 'what might you do with this insight?' Perhaps the difference between problem-solving and problem-management lies here: the former looks for solutions, the latter for goals to be achieved. In the sphere of emotions it is often the latter approach which is more realistic.

The problem-management approach is now clearly visible. When a goal has been identified, it has to be carried through. The next question therefore is, 'how are you going to do it?'

The questions (Tschudin, 1995, p. 56) just mentioned are very broad, and can be used with many other models. They can also be used as a model on their own for helping in either short or long-term helping situations. Yet they need never be asked in this way at all, because there are many ways of marking the phases through which a client passes when being helped by counselling. In this case they may merely be an *aide-mémoire*.

All the methods of helping and counselling are concerned first and foremost with the client or patient. They are therefore 'client-centred'. This word, however, is now being used for a particular approach, based on the work of Carl Rogers.

The *client-centred approach* (Rogers, 1961) was developed by Rogers, who can be regarded as the 'father' of counselling. Although his approach to helping is very soundly based in theory and practice, much of his appeal was a personal one. He was a man of great charisma, and it often seemed as if his presence alone was helpful to his clients. It is therefore not surprising that the hallmark of client-centred work is 'to help the client to become a self-accepted, insightful and fully functional individual' (Jones, 1990). This is achieved with the characteristics of warmth, non-judgemental attitude and empathy. The emphasis in this model is on the present, rather than on unconscious material from the past.

Rogers moved from first describing *client*-centred therapy to later referring to it as *person*-centred therapy. He was always concerned that the relationship between client and therapist (or counsellor or helper) is important and even crucial. Every writer and teacher on counselling is concerned with the relationship, which should be formal yet also informal, close but not oppressive, satisfactory to both but not dependent, equal but not 'matey'. Campbell (1984) described the relationships which nurses have with patients as 'skilled companionship', and this can also apply in the setting between helper and client.

According to Campbell, the *relationship* which nurses enjoy most is one of 'limited friendship with those patients who co-operate' (Campbell, 1984, p. 48). It is not overstating the case to say that this also applies generally to most helping relationships.

Campbell describes this skilled companionship as 'a closeness which is not sexually stereotyped; it implies movement and change; it expresses mutuality; and it requires commitment, but within defined limits' (Campbell, 1984, p. 49). This is very close to the ideal of empathy, which also demands closeness but not identity, helps the other to move and change without being overbearing, and often needs a long commitment – especially in any in-depth counselling. Empathy has sometimes been described as 'walking in the other's shoes', but this implies pushing the other out of his or her shoes. It is more correct to say that empathy allows a person to walk alongside another, becoming aware of what it is like for that other person to walk in his or her shoes and communicating this to him or her, so that he or she can eventually see whether the shoes need to be changed, and if so what should be worn instead.

Companionship is immediately associated with the image of a journey: the two people are on a journey together for a while, also knowing that the journey will eventually end. The word companion stems from the Latin *'com'* (with) and *'panis'* (bread). Thus the companion is someone who shares bread with another. This reinforces the idea that at the beginning of a helping process some physical assistance often has to be given. It also points to the image of the helper as someone who has something which the other needs and which is freely shared. Moreover, the image of the one 'with bread' is also the image of the nurse as nourisher.

Images convey some truth, but rarely represent the whole truth. Thus the image of the skilled companion was applied to nursing by Campbell (1984), and is here borrowed to be used for helpers in counselling situations as well. Inevitably, a counsellor is someone who is close, who shares and who encourages. However, he or she must also be able to challenge, to confront with reality, and to warn. To a client this may appear to be like a withdrawal.

This brings us back to the symbol of the nurse: the symbol of the good nurse who may be elusive, and the shadow or negative symbol of the nurse who withholds and withdraws. Before it is realistic to concentrate again on these symbols, the question of who is or can be a counsellor should be addressed.

Those who are *counsellors* in health care may be wearing a number of hats. Most nurses have some injunction in their job descriptions to counsel patients or clients and colleagues as and when necessary. Very often they will have had little training for this aspect of their work, and therefore might do it with apprehension or even suspicion. However, given the above description of the difference between counselling and using counselling skills, it is clear that anyone with some training should be able to help another person by means of counselling skills. Only when there is an agreement or contract for counselling does the person need to possess more than basic skills. Yet many highly skilled people have never taken a course in counselling and, conversely, many people who have taken courses are using the skills of counselling far from effectively.

It is right that there should be untrained people using their basic human skills to help others. It is also right that nurses use their perhaps limited counselling skills if and when called upon to do so. And it is right that fully trained counsellors should also be working as nurses and using their skills and training when appropriate. Those people can often be the centre of an unofficial support service, which nurses trust because there is no vested interest. However, such people should not be taken advantage of by employers. Employers have a duty to support their staff, and this should be done officially, with everyone knowing who the counsellor is and how they can have access to this person. Many hospitals and districts have full-time counsellors for their staff, but many do not. If a member of staff, such as a nurse or social worker, fulfils the role on a part-time basis, then this must also be clear. Such a person needs to be qualified and trained as a counsellor.

Mention needs to be made of the fact that any counselling service must be confidential, and employers should not have access to the records of the service, other than to simple statistical figures of attendance.

Those whose job is to counsel will also abide by the British Association for Counselling (BAC) *Code of Ethics and Practice for Councellors* (1990). This means that practitioners have regular *supervision* from a recognized supervisor. Those people who are using counselling skills as part of their main job or profession are not obliged to have supervision, but should be strongly encouraged to seek it. Counselling is demanding and can be relieving as well as damaging. When supervision is available, people are more likely to use their counselling skills and therefore feel more satisfied as individuals and also with the care given.

It is in helping others that counsellors become aware of the deeper dimensions of life which often rule behaviour. Counsellors will therefore need to have some knowledge of psychology, and to be familiar with the language and images of symbols. They will have to help their clients to make sense of material which is often only recognized in pictures, rather than in clear concepts. Counsellors working in health care therefore need to be able to recognize and interpret symbols such as that of the nurse used in this chapter. By their very nature, symbols are never completely understood or exhaustively explained, and it is therefore clear that any supervision should be helpful for exploring not only this, but other symbols too. Thus both the positive and the shadow side of this and other images can be described, used and applied.

Can the emotional cost be paid?

At the end of this chapter it is necessary to draw the various strands together and consider whether the emotional cost can be addressed with the various systems of support outlined.

Nobody would dispute that those who give care to others also need care for themselves. Yet it is still said of colleagues that 'she had to have counselling', implying that this is unfortunate and that this person is less worthy of being a nurse than others who have no similar need. At the NASS conference on 4 May 1994 the participants of one discussion group were quite adamant that students and staff had to change the culture in which such remarks could be made. They felt that they were doing this by showing solidarity with any member of staff who was receiving support, and making it clear to management that such people 'are OK'. The more they supported each other informally, the more they were also likely to have their own needs supported. Those who had faced needs and crises and worked through them were more respected than those who tried to brazen it out and then became hardened. They felt that it is not right to teach students to care holistically if the teachers do not include themselves in the model. They were concerned that their teachers exhibited split personalities by advocating one way of caring for patients and another for nurses. Indeed, this showed them that the shadow of the archetype of the nurse is alive and well, and stalking the schools and colleges of nursing.

The archetype of the nurse is one who nourishes, cares and mothers. However, among nurses it is usually the shadow who is more evident: the nurse who refuses to care, who does not heal and who keeps the person sick. The symbol describes an unconscious state, but it seems clear after the descriptions of the available support that this negative symbol dominates much of the nursing culture today. It is perhaps just because it is a symbol and unconscious that it is so elusive and also so destructive. Nurses have tried to change the culture by various means, such as the introduction of research and Project 2000, having a code of professional conduct, public accountability and expanding the role of nurses into independence. These are all attempts to slay the dragon of refusal to care and heal. If nurses were able to be entirely positive about themselves, they would no longer need to feel badly treated by their medical colleagues and 'the system'. They would no longer be the handmaidens who keep themselves in that position by identifying with a symbol which gives them power. When nurses can face the fact that they gain enormous power by keeping their profession and the culture of health care 'sick', then they will in fact be able to face the positive symbol of the nurse and begin to care realistically. Perhaps the recognition of a difference between guilt and constructive remorse might be helpful here.

When nurses realize that they personally and collectively need care, then they face the symbol of being nourished. When they become true companions of themselves, then they can also be companions to their patients and clients.

Giving and receiving support is more than just a meeting of two people; in that meeting there is a wider and deeper dimension – that of the symbol.

The emotional cost of feelings of anger, guilt and shame is also reflected in the unconscious. When the feelings are addressed, the unconscious ground shifts and the person who is helped comes closer to the symbolic understanding of the needs expressed through the feelings. In this way, every nurse who is helped and supported contributes to the shift in the culture which holds on tightly to a destructive force. By supporting and being supported we are helping not only ourselves but also the whole ethos of caring.

The emotional cost can indeed be measured in days of sickness and absence from work, and in billions of pounds lost to industry. It can also be measured symbolically in the nurses and health carers who are healthier and more fulfilled human beings because they have contributed to a culture which is holistic in the sense that it can integrate the conscious and the unconscious, the visible and the invisible, the tangible and its shadow. Then perhaps the economy, effectiveness and efficiency need no longer undermine knowledge, care and understanding: they will no longer be harmful, but tools in the nurses' hands.

Appendix I – A Charter for Staff Support. Reprinted with permission of NASS, the National Association for Staff Support.

Address of NASS:
NASS Central Office
9 Caradon Close
Woking GU21 3DU
Telephone: 01483 771 599

A Charter for
Staff Support

for staff in the health care services

Printed for the National Association for Staff Support
by the Royal College of Nursing

October 1992

A Charter for Staff Support

*for staff at all levels in the
health care and social services*

This Charter has been prepared by a group of organisations which are concerned with promoting good support practices for staff in the health care and social services.

It is intended as a guide for health authorities and any other organisations which employ staff to provide a caring service.

It sets out employers' responsibilities and the rights and responsibilities of all staff involved.

It provides a statement on the commitment required to maintain desirable standards for all aspects of staff support provision.

What is staff support?

Personal health care is often stressful, and over a period of time staff may become worn out or burnt out. Staff support helps those who care for others to be fully effective in their service. It recognises that the people who care are a most important resource.

■ Staff support involves more than incorporating recognised support systems, or bringing in a service at a time of crisis. Although these things are very important, staff support also involves the creation of a caring and healthy working environment and a culture which is an integral part of every institutional setting.

■ It ensures that a variety of support mechanisms are available.

■ It assists individuals to recognise stressful situations and to be aware of their own responses to stress and recognise their limitations.

■ It enables staff carers to acknowledge sensitivity and to develop and use their own coping mechanisms and strengths.

■ It turns supervision into a recreative process which encourages, teaches and improves the quality of professional work.

■ It fosters a management structure which ensures that individuals are valued.

Staff support recognises that people are a most valuable and valued resource and therefore the need for support is seen as legitimate and acceptable – in short, *a good thing.*

Why is staff support necessary?

All staff working in any kind of health care services are human beings with rights, needs and feelings just like other citizens, but they are subjected to specific pressures generated by the stressful nature of their work. Therefore they are entitled to have these conditions recognised and adequate provision made for their relief.

The consequences of occupational stress are known to be very serious for both employing authorities and staff. The costs are high in terms of staff turnover, sickness and work performance, and a continuing drain on valuable resources, thus having far reaching effects on the quality of patient care.

The personal effects on the individual can be devastating in terms of both physical and mental health.

Much of this damage can be prevented by:

Recognising that stress exists

Acknowledging the need for support

Educating staff in prevention and management of stress

Providing adequate support services

Creating a caring culture in the workplace

Promoting good staff support practices throughout the system.

There are many ways of accomplishing the

provision of good staff support through existing services such as:

- Occupational health services
- Counselling services
- Chaplaincy departments
- In-service training courses
- 'Time out' arrangements
- Peer support groups
- Good communications
- Educational departments
- Good management
- A good environment

Work related issues are very often dealt with by professional organisations, unions or occupational health services. These can also play an important part in promoting a healthy and safe working environment and contributing to staff support provision.

Policy principles

The following general principles are an essential part of any national or local policy:

- Staff in health care services have individual rights to be valued and respected just as any other citizens have.
- Staff who are cared for provide the best quality of service; where there is inadequate care and support, staff will

show high sickness, absenteeism and wastage rates.

■ Staff are a valued and expensive resource. It makes good sense to maintain their fitness and capacity to give a good service in the interests of their personal job satisfaction and of maintaining the quality of patient care.

■ A range of integrated services together with a general ethos of care is an essential provision. Also recognition of the nature of stress and of the need for emotional support in the workplace at all times is important.

■ Identifying who is responsible for providing a stated policy, both nationally and locally, is necessary for coordination in all workplaces.

Implementing national policies at local level

Given the acceptance of these general principles:

■ Each authority or organisation is responsible for drafting its own policy on good staff support practices, in the context of local needs and existing resources. All staff should know about it.

■ Employers are responsible for ensuring that each member of staff has a copy of the policy and services provided and a statement of the conditions they can expect.

■ Staff are entitled to recognition and consideration of their personal needs and to have access on demand to adequate support in their workplace. Such provision includes access to personal development training, as distinct from professional training.

■ Staff are entitled to have access to immediate debriefing facilities following any traumatic situation and to have such facilities available as part of a normal daily service.

■ Managers at all levels need to be educated about counselling skills and to be sensitive to staff needs so they can ensure that the appropriate support is available.

■ Staff need to be aware that it is acceptable to seek help. They need assurance that counselling available through professional service is completely confidential in all respects, and in accordance with approved ethical principles.

■ Listening and communication skills are part of the basic tools required by all professional staff and their use can be encouraged to enhance support at local level within any team.

■ Training in recognition of the signs of stress in individuals, coping mechanisms and stress management is essential for all managers.

■ A satisfactory working environment in all respects is a vital part of staff support. This includes facilities for 'time out' after stressful periods, and for sustaining adequate staff provision, both in numbers and skills mix, so that standards of service can be maintained without compromising individual professional practice.

■ Staff need to know the identity of the person to whom they can turn, with the assurance that they will be heard, if any of these standards and good practices are not maintained.

Rights and responsibilities

Where there are rights there are also responsibilities for both staff and employers.

All staff have the right to expect:

■ Staff support provisions as outlined in this Charter.

■ Employers to provide reasonable protection from violence in the workplace.

■ Opportunity to participate as appropriate in decision making.

■ Communication and adequate information about proposed changes in conditions.

■ Respect for their right to withdraw from participation in procedures which are against their conscience or beliefs, while maintaining their responsibility to provide patient care.

Individual members of staff can assume responsibility for improving some aspects of staff support within their own immediate working environment through:

■ **Recognising** the effects of stress on themselves and colleagues

■ **Offering** personal support and encouragement to colleagues

■ **Offering** thanks and appreciation where appropriate

■ **Considering** ways in which their own environment can be improved

■ **Knowing** exactly what local facilities are available

■ **Knowing** what their own professional organisation can do to help

■ **Knowing** the arrangements for reporting failure to provide their basic individual rights

Managers and employers also have rights as well as responsibilities. They too are human and need adequate support. Therefore they have the right to expect:

■ That staff in return will give loyal service and provide only the highest standards of patient care

■ Respect, support and appreciation from colleagues where appropriate

■ Access to adequate support provision for their own needs.

They are responsible for:

■ Promoting, establishing and maintaining good staff support practices and provisions within their organisation, as outlined in this Charter, thus creating and facilitating a caring culture.

The preparation of this Charter has been coordinated by the National Association for Staff Support for staff within the health services. Acknowledgements are due to the following individuals, who formed an ad hoc advisory group.

Chairman: Rev David Stoter	Co-ordinator of Chaplains, Nottingham Hospitals, Chairman of NASS Council
Grace Owen	General Secretary, NASS
Meg Barham	Staff Counsellor, St Thomas' Hospital
Professor Brandon	Secretary, Counselling Service for Sick Doctors
David Charles-Edwards	Charles-Edwards Associates
Dr Graham Curtis-Jenkins	Director, Primary Care Trust
Ann Good	Formerly Head of Oasis
Christine Hancock	General Secretary, Royal College of Nursing
John Maher	Senior Welfare Adviser, Nurses' Welfare Service
Audrey Newsome	Chairman of UK Forum for Organisational Health
Isobel Palmer	Information and Publications Manager, British Association for Counselling
Colin Somerville	Senior Counsellor, CHAT, Royal College of Nursing
Verena Tschudin	Member of UK Forum for Organisational Health

Acknowledgements are also due to the RCN for their assistance with production facilities.

Further copies of this Charter may be obtained by sending an appropriately stamped addressed envelope (A5 size) to NASS Central Office.

References

Barber P (1993) Developing the 'person' of the professional carer. In Hinchliff SM, Norman SE and Schober JE (eds) *Nursing Practice and Health Care*, 2nd edn, pp. 344–73. Edward Arnold, London.
British Association for Counselling (1990) *Code of Ethics and Practice for Counsellors*. British Association for Counselling, Rugby.
Campbell AV (1984) *Moderated Love*. SPCK, London.
Carkhuff RR (1987) *The Art of Helping*, 6th edn. Human Resource Development Press, Amherst, MA.
Chetwynd T (1982) *A Dictionary of Symbols*. Paladin, London.
Dryden W (1994) *Overcoming Guilt*. Sheldon Press, London.
Egan G (1994) *The Skilled Helper*, 5th edn. Brooks/Cole, Belmont, CA.
Jones C (1990) All you ever wanted to know about counselling. *Nursing Times* 86, 55–8.
Jung CG (1964) *Man and His Symbols*. Aldus Books Ltd, republished in 1978 by Pan Books Ltd, London.

Kershaw B (1994) Professionalism and professional qualifications. In Tschudin V (ed.) *Ethics: Professional Issues*, pp. 61–83. Scutari, London.

National Association for Staff Support (1992a) *A Charter for Staff Support*. National Association for Staff Support, Woking.

National Association for Staff Support (1992b) *The Costs of Stress and the Costs and Benefits of Stress Management*. National Association for Staff Support, Woking.

Nelson-Jones R (1993) *Practical Counselling and Helping Skills*. Cassell, London.

Nursing Standard (1994) News item: hospice nurses with support less likely to use 'blocking'. Nursing Standard 8, 14.

Owen G (1993) *'Taking the Strain': Stress, Coping Mechanisms and Support Systems for Professional Carers. Literature Review*, 5th edn. National Association for Staff Support, Woking.

Parry G (1990) *Coping with Crises*. British Psychological Society in association with Routledge (London), Leicester.

Rogers CR (1961) *On Becoming a Person*. Constable, London.

Smith P (1992) *The Emotional Labour of Nursing*. Macmillan, Basingstoke.

Stewart W (1992) *An A–Z of Counselling Theory and Practice*. Chapman and Hall, London.

Tschudin V (1995) *Counselling Skills for Nurses*, 4th edn. Baillière Tindall, London.

United Kingdom Central Council for Nursing, Midwifery and Health Visiting (UKCC) (1995) *Eight Factsheets: 'PREP and You'*. UKCC, London.

Wheeler H and Riding R (1994) Occupational stress in general nurses and midwives. *British Journal of Nursing* 3, 527–34.

Wood (1990) Psychotherapy: a counselling success. *Occupational Health*, October, 292–6.

Further reading

Mackay L (1993) *Conflicts in Care: Medicine and Nursing*. London. Chapman and Hall, London.

Roach MS (1992) *The Human Act of Caring: A Blueprint for the Health Professions*, revised edn. Canadian Hospital Association Press, Ottawa.

Watson J (ed.) (1994) *Applying the Art and Science of Human Caring*. National League for Nursing Press, New York.

9

Care costs: towards a critical understanding of care

Pam Smith and Ellen Agard

Nurses are predominantly female, and for the most part are holding down two social roles and functions, one as paid employees of the health-care system, and another as home- and house-keepers. These two demanding roles, together with the legacy of the politics that gender entails, mean that for most nurses their working life can be stressful and excessively demanding. Despite this, the majority of nurses want to be caring; they are aware of the price that caring in these circumstances can demand, they want to be competent and knowledgeable, and they wish to be culturally sensitive to the needs of their patients. They are dimly aware of what the arts can offer to promote these caring strategies, and they may even faintly recall the roots of their own nursing culture and the historical traditions of their profession. However, this may not be enough. This final chapter will look at nurses who care, and at the price that they are prepared to pay in order to be effective and relevant to their patient and client groups. Yet unless nurses start to view their nursing care in a wider socio-economic and political context, they may find themselves no longer the core and most significant providers of nursing care. In any attempt to examine the nature of nursing care realistically, however, careful attention needs to be paid to the research methodologies used to justify nursing's claims and demonstrate nursing's concerns. The very process of demonstrating the need for expert care and the value of nursing needs to be undertaken with an academic honesty and political astuteness that allows for justice and an equal voice for all of the disfranchised and vulnerable. Without this wisdom and compassion, both nurses and their patients may become the losers in the new health-care scenario.

Introduction

In both the USA and UK, the delivery of health care is being restructured. Although the health-care systems are very different, both are faced with the need to contain costs, to deliver services more efficiently, and to reduce waste. Nurses in both health-care systems are experiencing similar stresses as the conditions of their work change. In this chapter, we reflect on these changes, situating them in their social and economic context and exploring their significance. Our method is anecdotal and narrative, and our insights are derived from our own observations and practice in nursing and nursing research, and from our dialogue, in which the similarities of the UK and the US health-care systems impress us more forcibly than the differences.

While visiting the USA to study health-care reform, one of the authors was able to follow an urban public-health nurse on her rounds. As our paper took shape, we found ourselves turning to these visits to illustrate graphically the needs that nurses try to address, and the pressures that they face in their care-giving work. We begin our analysis with two vignettes drawn from these public-health visits, and we present these vignettes for two reasons. First, they illustrate the growing demand for services and the shrinking resources being placed on helping professions today; the stresses faced by the public-health nurse are similar to those faced by social workers, teachers and hospital nurses. Secondly, they raise the following questions which we address in our paper: what is the nature of care, who provides care in our society, and why?

Following the vignettes, we analyse care on two levels: as work and as labour. Work denotes what nurses do – their skills, tasks and productivity, both tangible and intangible. Nursing work is an extension of the caring work done in the private or domestic sphere, largely by women. Labour denotes the selling of nursing work for a wage, in the public or private sectors. Nursing labour is a product which can be expropriated, exploited, and influenced by market forces. We contend that it is necessary to understand nursing on both levels in order to provide a full account of nursing practice.

First, we draw on the literature in order to examine the nature of care-giving work, the experience of doing it, and how it is learned and validated. We distinguish between lay and professional care, and focus on the professional care-giving provided by the registered nurse. We ask why nurses find it difficult to provide a meaningful account of their work outside their own professional group. This enquiry requires us to examine the marginalization of nursing in the division of labour of health-care delivery.

Next, we analyse care as labour, drawing on feminist and sociological literature in order to scrutinize the social arrangements and assumptions which shape care-giving in both the public and the domestic spheres (and the private and public health-care sectors). This literature highlights the role of the nurse in the provision of health and social services and the vulnerability of nursing and care to market vagaries. We identify some underlying assumptions on which care is based – predominantly women's work, which is gendered, marginal and of low social priority.

Finally, we offer a critical theory of nursing practice in which we deconstruct the phenomenon of caring in order to challenge some basic assumptions of nursing theory and relocate it in its social and political context. Specifically, we challenge nursing's unexamined commitment to an ethos of care, suggesting that it legitimates the appropriation of women's work in both the paid and unpaid sectors, and that the true social costs of caring work are obscured when women carry the responsibility for caring without adequate recognition or recompense. We conclude by recommending critical research methodology which integrates an analysis of care both as work and as labour, and which gives voice to front-line nurses.

Vignettes: care on the front line

A public-health nurse makes her first visit to an African-American man with HIV infection who has just returned from the hospital following an episode of severe illness. He is weak and debilitated, trying to make sense of his illness and to plan for his future. Self-employed, no longer working, and without health insurance, his greatest concern is how he will pay for his health care. The public-health nurse advises him on how to apply for Medicaid (state medical insurance) to cover his health care. She explains his medications, tells him how to avoid infections, and discusses strategies for surviving and coping with his life-threatening illness. The public-health nurse's visit has a visible impact: her client looks more cheerful, and is reassured that he can rely upon regular visits and telephone contact.

The public-health nurse's next visit is to a young single mother and her 2-month-old baby. This is not a 'routine' baby visit – the mother is participating in a drug rehabilitation programme. Her questions reveal the obstacles she faces and the anxiety she feels. Will her baby's development be impaired because of her addiction? Is the baby developing normally now? The public-health nurse also asks questions. Is the baby feeding well? Does the mother have enough social and financial support to care for her baby? Again, the public-health nurse's visit is encouraging and reassuring.

During both visits we can see how the public-health nurse listens, responds to her clients and gives positive encouragement to their considerable efforts to deal with life and death issues. She is prepared to cover a range of problems from lack of health-care coverage to substance abuse and to give practical suggestions about all aspects from diet to finance. Her professional training and experience have prepared her to deal with this range of problems, but she does not respond without personal cost.

At the end of the day, we can see how her energy and enthusiasm have drained away to be replaced by exhaustion. She explains that most of her clients these days have complex histories and needs, like the people we visited. 'Routine' visits to promote the health of new mothers and babies, school children or senior citizens have virtually disappeared from her caseload. With tight resources, only the most extreme cases qualify to stay on the books.

In a tense economic atmosphere of recession and competition, public services and benefits are being pared to the bone, with only the most needy and complex finding their way on to the public-health nurse's caseload. The eligibility criteria are stringent and benefits are limited, as her clients have found. For example, the new mother in drug rehabilitation gets assistance from a federally funded nutrition support programme for Women, Infants and Children (WIC), and could not manage without the food vouchers, yet finds them insufficient for her child's needs. The man with HIV infection meets the eligibility requirements for Medicaid, but will be covered only for a limited set of benefits from a limited number of providers. Living alone and struggling to shop and cook for himself, he relies on food programmes such as Meals on Wheels. Thus part of the public-health nurse's job is to connect her clients to a patchwork of voluntary and public services, helping them to find and access the services for which they qualify. Under financial constraints, there are fewer services to go round, and the clients who qualify for them are sicker and more needy.

What do these vignettes tell us about care?

In reflecting on these vignettes, we notice several factors which affect the work done by the public-health nurse.

First, the nature of her work is shaped by economic and bureaucratic forces beyond her control. Administrators make decisions based on financial and organizational criteria. Direct-services providers are seldom involved in these decisions; both their work and their insights are undervalued. Thus the public-health nurse working on the front-line of health-care delivery finds her work increasingly stressful as she tries to meet high levels of need with ever decreasing resources of time, energy and money. The pressures and dilemmas she confronts are not unique to nursing, but are common to other caring professions. Individuals in these professions try to close the gap between what is needed and what can be provided. They take responsibility for clients, patients or students, but they control neither the demand for services nor the resources available to meet those demands.

Despite the title of *public*-health nurse, much of the 'public' is unaware of the work she does. It takes place on an interface between public and private, publicly funded and organized but carried out within the privacy of clients' homes, away from the public gaze. Her work is directly seen and valued only by clients and their families. Because of its low visibility, it is not recognized or valued either by society as a whole, or by colleagues and researchers such as ourselves.

The status of her clients contributes to the invisibility and undervaluing of the public-health nurse's work. Often client status is a critical factor in determining how human service work is valued and funded. In the UK, for example, services for the elderly, disabled and mentally ill have traditionally been labelled the 'Cinderella' services because of the double jeopardy of low status and chronic underfunding. In the USA, and increasingly in the UK, public-health nursing services tend to serve those who are socially and economically marginalized by gender, race, class, sexual orientation or employment status. The problems of HIV infection and drug addiction seen in our vignettes are stigmatized, stereotyped and socially sanctioned as symbols of social breakdown.

Client status can also affect the status of those who work with the clients. Nurses who specialize in mental health or long-term care get less recognition than those who specialize in acute care. Some of the stigma attached to such negatively perceived groups as sex workers or illegal drug users carries over to the researchers who study them (Renzetti and Lee, 1992). Similarly, the public-health nurse's work is under-recognized and undervalued in part because of the low status of her clients.

The vignettes also illustrate how hard it is to quantify the care work done by the public-health nurse, and how she contributes to 'the material and emotional upkeep' of her clients (Juteau and Laurin, 1989). Her contributions, particularly to her clients' emotional well-being, are difficult to convey on official documents, and their social and individual outcomes are difficult to measure. We cannot 'prove' that, as a direct result of the public-health nurse's intervention, a mother and baby will have more stable and healthy lives, or that a man will find his life-threatening illness less lonely and more tolerable. In part this is because emotional well-being is not easily quantified, but it is also partly because contributions to emotional well-being are subsumed under nurturing attitudes and activities which have traditionally been associated with women's roles or women's nature.

It is no accident that the public-health nurse is a woman. The majority of front-line workers in the caring professions are women. Of approximately 2.1 million hospital and community nurses in the USA, 97 per cent are women. Of 3.7 million teachers, 73 per cent are women, and of 527 000 social workers, 68 per cent are women (cited in Gordon, 1991b). Similar trends in Europe show a predominance of women in these professional groups. In the UK, for example, 404 000 nurses and midwives account for over half of the health service's total work force, and 90 per cent are women (cited in Beardshaw and Robinson, 1990).

In addition, being a paid care provider is only the tip of the iceberg. Many women are involved throughout their domestic lives in a 'cycle of care', tending children, partners and sick, disabled and/or elderly relatives (Ungerson, 1983). Surveys show that the majority of chronically ill and disabled people in the USA and Europe are cared for at home by female kin (Ward, 1993). The young woman in our second vignette could not have survived without the financial and emotional support of her own mother. Thus women find themselves as the principal care-givers in both the domestic and public spheres. For the public-health nurse, public and private merge. As she provides paid work in the domestic setting, she draws on both her professional duties and her personal attitudes and orientation; only the former is recognized and compensated.

Some feminists have been reluctant to emphasize the value of caring because they fear its traditional association with women will make the latter even more vulnerable to exploitation (Gordon 1991a). For this reason, our discussion of care goes beyond an analysis of the nature of care-giving as women's work and commitment to examine the social context in which caring takes place.

Nursing care: work and commitment

Nurses represent the largest occupational group in health care, and carry a major responsibility for meeting our health care needs, yet nursing has received limited scholarly attention outside its own discipline.[9.1] While the nursing profession is becoming more vocal and more active politically, we struggle to account for the role of nurses in health-care delivery, and the nature and value of the work that we do, in ways that are convincing to those outside the profession. In many ways, nurses are silent and invisible, and their work is taken for granted and poorly understood.

Ann Oakley, an eminent British sociologist and feminist, confesses that it took a life-threatening illness to alert her to nurses' contribution to health care. She writes:

> In a fifteen-year career as a sociologist studying medical services, I confess that I have been particularly blind to the contribution made by nurses to health care. Indeed, over a period of some months spent observing in a large London hospital, I hardly noticed nurses at all. I took their presence for granted (much as, I imagine, the doctors and patients did) – and the character of the nurse's role in no way impressed itself on me.
>
> (Oakley, 1984, p. 24)

What caused Oakley to change her mind? Following a diagnosis of cancer of the tongue she was admitted to hospital for radon implants. Because of the radiation hazard she was placed in a single room under protective isolation. Anyone entering the room had to wear a gown, mask and gloves, maintain their distance from her, and stay for not longer than five minutes. On a day when Oakley was feeling particularly dispirited, a nurse noticed her mood and sat with her for twenty minutes, disregarding the need for protective clothing in order to maintain close contact. Oakley never saw her again, but attributes her survival to that nurse's understanding and kindness.[9.2]

In recent decades a rich body of nursing scholarship has been devoted to describing, analysing and validating the practice of nursing. In this literature, the language of care is so pervasive, and the association between nursing work and caring attitudes and actions so explicit, that even a brief excursion into the nursing literature yields a wealth of information about care and its distinctive place in nursing. This literature views care as a basic human need and capacity, and as a system of learned skills and practices. Underlying these aspects of care is an understanding of care as a relationship and moral commitment. Nursing responds to basic human needs for care in a skilled manner, but ideally this response is guided by a caring attitude.

In her study of British student nurses, Smith (1992) found that they identified the 'little things' or caring gestures as being important to their elderly patients. Tasks such as giving injections, bathing and toileting were performed with care. Caring attitudes were expressed through activities such as adjusting hearing aids, helping elderly patients to choose library books, or taking them on outings. Smith analyses care work as involving both tasks and emotional style. On the one hand, tasks are performed with a caring attitude; on the other, caring attitudes are expressed through caring activities.[93]

In her philosophical work on care, Noddings (1984) describes attitude and action as being intrinsically connected. Action on behalf of another is not caring unless it is guided by an attitude of care; at the same time, an attitude of care is insufficient without caring action. This intrinsic connection is prominent in the nursing literature, where nursing is presented as a practice which combines distinctive knowledge and skills with a distinctive attitude or moral orientation towards care.

For Leininger (1990), an anthropologist and nursing scholar, care is a basic human need and capacity, and 'the central phenomenon and essence of nursing'. While nursing is but one expression of human caring, its 'care knowledge and skills' and its organized approach to care-giving can be taught and learned, making it a distinctive discipline or profession. What makes nursing distinctive for Leininger is the centrality of care as a moral value and commitment.

For Benner and Wrubel (1989), nursing researchers and educators, caring is a form of expertise and a set of skills and practice which are learned, developed and transmitted. They describe nursing as a practice or a strategy which responds to specific human situations with practical knowledge and skill. For Benner and Wrubel, as for Leininger, nursing expertise in recognizing and responding to human need is guided by values of human relationship and commitment.

These efforts to define nursing work contribute to our understanding of what caring work entails. Caring work involves both tasks and emotional style – tasks performed with an attitude of care, and an attitude of care expressed in some form of caring activity. In an attempt to define and validate what nurses do, the nursing profession claims this blend of action and attitude as their distinctive territory. However, despite considerable efforts to identify what is unique about nursing practice, the nursing profession has been unable to claim a territory which belongs to nursing alone. Instead, the scope of nursing practice, and therefore the work that nurses do, expands and contracts in response to external demands. In order to reduce the costs of providing health care, more highly skilled tasks commonly performed by junior physicians or therapists can be passed on to nurses, and the less skilled tasks commonly performed by nurses can be passed on to less highly skilled personnel, or to relatives.[94] We are left with an understanding of nursing work which remains vulnerable to exploitation as nursing labour, which we shall examine in the next section.

Care as labour

Nursing work is a product which can be sold and exploited, that is, wages can be set according to economic forces rather than according to the full value of the work or the cost to the person performing it. As nursing labour, the services which nurses perform are shaped by changes in the social and economic context within which nursing work is performed.

We suggest that, since emotions, feelings, communication and relationships are so central to nursing discourse, the notion of emotional labour provides one way of understanding what nurses provide that is not fully recognized or fully compensated.

Our concept of emotional labour is drawn from Hochschild's study of flight attendants, within which she developed the idea of emotional labour as 'the induction or suppression of feeling in order to sustain in others a sense of being cared for in a convivial safe place' (Hochschild, 1983, p. 7). Emotional labour is sold for a wage and has exchange value.

In the study referred to above, Smith describes the emotional work nurses do in helping patients to cope with illness and hospitalization, explores how that work can be done or not done according to its context, and raises issues about the gendered nature of nursing work. Smith found that care included the emotional labour involved in setting a caring attitude or caring atmosphere created by the ward sister (head nurse).

Emotional labour as a component of care is gendered. At the time of Hochschild's study in the early 1980s, she estimated that over half of all working women had jobs that call for emotional labour. Flight attendants, like nurses, are predominantly women, only 15 per cent being men. As both male and female flight attendants undertake the same work in the same place, Hochschild suggests that 'any difference in work experience is due to gender'.

With the growth of the service sector during the 1970s and 1980s, communication and encounter have become the central work relationship on which the quality of service is judged. For example, passengers judged the quality of the airline by the emotional style of its personnel. Airline companies recognized the profit implications of providing a quality service, trained their flight attendants to do emotional labour, and paid them relatively high wages. Emotional labour was thus transformed into a commodity which by its visibility would attract business.

In nursing during this time period the nursing process was introduced as a philosophy and work method which raised the profile of emotional care by emphasizing people and communication, rather than tasks. However, unlike the airline industry, which paid flight attendants for their emotional labour, the emotional rewards of nursing are still seen as supplementing the financial ones. A 1990 national recruitment advertisement in the UK reassures prospective nurses that, although they are unlikely to be attracted to the job for financial reasons, they will be well paid for their skills. The predominant message is clearly that nursing, as one of the 'most emotionally satisfying professions', offers more than financial rewards. This message does not differ substantially from that in an early edition of the *American Journal of Nursing* (Turkoski, 1992), which suggests that women should never expect the same wages as men because providing a service is more important than renumeration.

In the case of nursing, these skills are blended with technical expertise and a psychosocial, emotional, ethical and moral commitment to care. According to Ray (1987), this unique blend of skills was apparent in critical-care nursing, which 'displayed both human and technocratic aspects and was seen as an ethical and moral process' (Ray, 1987, p. 167). However, Hart (1991) saw nurses' multiple skills and their ability to cover for domestic and medical shortages as both their strength and their undoing. Their adaptability to changing situations was their strength, but in management terms this was also their undoing since it proved that nursing skills were 'unspecialized, interchangeable and easily transferable' (James, 1991, cited in Hart, 1991).

In the domestic sphere, a study of working couples with young children showed that it was predominantly women who managed the dual and complex task of balancing paid employment and family care (Hochschild, 1989). Hochschild's study shows how the tasks associated with the domestic sphere and the work of care in the public sphere are blended to keep women's work invisible and inadequately renumerated. It is convenient for women's domestic labour to be viewed in this way, because their complex but undervalued skills can be reproduced in the market-place at minimum financial cost. Just as women's management of complex domestic situations is neither visible nor valued by society, the adaptability of nurses is not seen as a skill.

According to Gordon (1991b), the consequences of women's work being invisible and undervalued are twofold. In addition to economic effects, women also suffer psychologically from lowered self-esteem and lack of self-confidence as a result of performing public and private tasks that at best are seen as inferior, and at worst are neither recognized nor rewarded.

An adequate account of care-giving must therefore include an analysis of both care as work and care as labour. It must also explain its gendered and marginalized nature.

Care and gender

In a recent discussion of gender and health care, Riska states that:

> It is hard to think of any other sector of the economy that is still as labour-intensive and segregated by gender as health care. The basis of the division rests on the medical profession's claim that it possesses a special knowledge.
>
> (Riska, 1993, p. 7)

This statement points to two significant features of nursing work. First, medicine lays claim to a special body of knowledge which differs from and is superior to nursing knowledge. Medical knowledge is seen as objective and scientific, and emanates from a 'male-stream' view of the world (Smith, 1992).[9.5] Nursing knowledge and skills have been shaped and controlled by this perspective (Freidson, 1970). Because of their gender, nurses have been cast as emotional experts by female doctors and nurses as well as by their male counterparts; part of their job is to manage emotions and interactions in order to keep things running smoothly in the health-care setting. This type of work has been called 'emotion management' (Hochschild, 1983) or 'sentimental work' (Strauss *et al.*, 1985). Doctors and nurses perform different kinds of sentimental work. Doctors use it to gain trust and co-operation in order to obtain information and perform procedures; nurses use it to provide explanations and comfort patients following medical interactions and procedures (Strauss *et al.*, 1985).

Secondly, nursing has historically been a women's profession, and the association between nursing and female gender persists, barely modified by the recent entry of men into the profession. Furthermore, the gender division of labour in health care has segregated men and women into different health-care compartments. The professional dominance of medicine has strategically blocked competition from predominantly female health professions such as nursing and midwifery (Freund and McGuire, 1991; Witz, 1992).[9.6]

In recent years, a number of sociological and feminist theories have been postulated to explain and analyse the gendered nature of women's domestic and paid work (Finch and Groves, 1983; Glazer, 1993). While a full exploration and assessment of these theories is beyond the scope of this chapter, they effectively challenge some of the stereotypes and assumptions surrounding women as 'natural' care-givers.

First, the division of roles and responsibilities by gender, and the perception that women's care-giving and emotion management are an expression of their nature, is associated with an imbalance of power. Historically, men have had greater access to the public sphere, greater social and economic rewards and greater power than women.[9.7] The effects of this imbalance of power may not be felt by individuals or groups, but it affects the structure of society in ways which oppress women (Dahlerup, 1987).[9.8]

Important indicators of structural oppression include segregation of work between the sexes (Dahlerup, 1987) and, citing Hartmann (1979), the servicing of men by women.

Secondly, the division between a domestic and a public sphere has been challenged; we cannot obtain a full account of women's oppression until we understand how their work in the domestic sphere and their paid employment in the public sphere are intimately and structurally related (Dahlerup, 1987). The oppression of women has roots in their confinement to the activities and responsibilities of the domestic sphere, but we need an account of women's work which recognizes not only their exclusion from the public sphere, but also the ways in which their participation in the public sphere is shaped and restricted by gender. The public sphere expands or contracts according to economics, and women take up the slack as both paid and unpaid care providers.[9.9]

Thus nursing work, a particular set of knowledge and skills, and nursing labour, a product sold for a wage, are shaped by women's social location and by the gender division of labour in health care. Both the scope of nursing practice and the value set on their work are largely outside their control.

Care, class and race

Although we have focused so far on the gendered nature of nursing, there are divisions in health care and in nursing that are based on characteristics other than gender. The public portrayal of nurses in UK recruitment literature and advertisements tends to portray them as female and white; only recently have males and non-white people begun to appear in the public images of nursing, despite their significant presence and contributions to the profession. Men and non-white people in nursing have suffered from harassment and discrimination, as well as from stereotyping.

For example, in the UK, the first men to enter the nursing profession were recruited into psychiatric nursing because of the need to restrain patients physically before the advent of psychotropic medication. Men who became nurses were often labelled as gay and seen as 'funny and effeminate', without any evidence to support this stereotype. On the other hand, any lesbian presence in nursing was subsumed under the 'battleaxe' stereotype (Salvage, 1985). Thus sexual orientation in nursing, as in society at large, has been a problematic and stigmatized category.

With regard to black nurses, one study (Baxter, 1988) shows how they were specifically recruited to undertake lower level training and channelled into specialties perceived as being less prestigious, such as care of elderly patients and people with learning disabilities. Their promotion prospects were also poorer than those of their white counterparts.

Smith's (1992) research, conducted in an élite teaching hospital in the early 1980s, confirms this view. She found that students were recruited to conform to a white, female middle-class image. Another study shows that the nursing work-force in a high-employment, high-wage area of England is predominantly white (Robinson, 1992).

Gender and race combine to produce an over-representation of white men at senior management level in nursing (Baxter, 1988, Robinson, 1992). Ten per cent of the nursing work-force are men, but this percentage increases significantly for senior managers in education and service (Gaze, 1987, cited in Beardshaw and Robinson, 1990; Robinson, 1992). Thus men predominate, even in a predominantly female occupation.

Role of nurses in health-care delivery

As the vignettes at the beginning of this chapter illustrate, nurses serve the underserved – the uninsured and the underprivileged. These groups are underserved in that public resources are not adequate to deal with the problems of poor housing, inadequate nutrition, violence and limited access to health care which they confront. Because the underserved are of low social priority, social arrangements are not altered in order to accommodate the nurses who serve them. Instead, nurses act as intermediaries between individuals and the limited social resources available to them.

Perspectives on social values, the common good, and individual and collective responsibilities vary widely. Historically, the UK has been more willing than the USA to subsidize social services with public funds; the differences in social-care arrangements in the USA and the UK reflect the underlying social values of each country. However, there is a shift in the UK towards emphasis on individual rather than state responsibility for the provision of welfare or care, and an associated shift from a service to a market ethos (Smith, 1996). In the USA, health-care restructuring indicates a commitment to competitive health care, with little attention being paid to the implications of this approach for health-care delivery.

The provision of welfare has a significant impact on women. The growth of the welfare state has led to an increase in women's involvement in paid caring work. The predominance of women in this sector of employment means that women carry a dual burden of care at home and at work (Waerness, 1987; Hochschild, 1989). The state relies on women's domestic labour to support the traditional household of male breadwinner (Finch and Groves, 1983; McIntosh, 1978, cited in Finch and Groves, 1983). Ironically, generous public support makes it possible for women to become financially independent of men while becoming financially dependent on the state instead (Dahlerup, 1987).

In the 1990s, health care, whether publicly or privately funded, is about reducing costs. Inevitably, nurses as the largest occupational group are used in a variety of ways to save money.

In the US privatized health-care systems, they may work on the telephone helplines of Health Maintenance Organizations in order to keep patients out of emergency rooms, they may answer telephone enquiries in response to advertisements for laser surgery and other hospital treatments, or they may be employed by health insurance companies to check claims before agreeing to reimburse treatments. They may be employed as clinical nurse specialists by pharmaceutical companies to administer and manage their products, e.g. by means of parenteral nutrition and intravenous drug therapy. A personal communication from an eminent nurse academic suggested a future role for nurses as 'brokers' of health care in order to achieve a better fit between needs and service and to keep costs down. Schroeder's (1993) description of a nurse-led service for people with HIV/AIDS demonstrated this approach. One way of making savings in the service was attributed to the formation of nurse–client partnerships which enabled clients to make the best and most effective use of services.

Until the current crisis in health-care costs, nurses were used in the US health-care industry to attract patients to their hospitals (compare with the example of flight attendants cited earlier). For example, during the 1980s, the 'Magnet' hospitals cited as representing some of the top management practices amongst US industry promoted primary nursing (one-to-one patient care from admission to discharge) as a means of improving nurse recruitment and patient satisfaction. Evidence suggested that patients chose those hospitals because of the quality of nursing offered (Kramer and Schmalenberg, 1988).

In the UK's relatively small but expanding private sector, the nurse has been used as an advertising image to encourage prospective patients to take out private health insurance. One leading company with its own network of private hospitals projects the following image. The smiling, uniformed nurse in pleasant hospital surroundings holds the patient's hand and joins in cheerful conversation with her family. The caption reads: 'Feel confident that when you or a member of your family need hospital treatment, you'll enjoy comfort, privacy and individual attention'. The language appears to be directed to a middle-class, élite clientele.

In the UK, however, the nurse's prime role has been in the public provision of care to the majority of the population rather than to the socially and economically marginalized, as in the USA. It is important to note, therefore, that the ideology informing the financing and organization of public-sector caring in the USA differs fundamentally from that in the UK, other countries of Western Europe and Canada. Gordon writes that: 'Where other industrialised nations have tempered the impersonality and ruthlessness of the marketplace with institutions that provide caring services to all citizens,' the American public is 'still skeptical of the notion that the purposes of government might include providing for human caring, community and collective action to achieve broad public good' (Gordon, 1991b, p. 20). The Clinton administration's attempt to revisit this notion with proposals for health-care reform was met with insurmountable political resistance; the result has been a rapid increase in the commercialization of health care in the USA.

In summary, nurses as the largest occupational group within health care are used by both public and private systems to promote a caring image which can help profits in good times and save costs during economic cutbacks. In the case of state provision they are used, like the public-health nurse in our vignettes, to meet the needs of complex groups who would otherwise fall through the net of diminishing resources. These examples illustrate how women in general and nurses in particular are dependent on market forces for their participation in the work-force.

Impact of market forces on women's participation in the work-force

From the specific example of nuns in Quebec, Juteau and Laurin make a general point about women in the labour market:

> On the paid labor market, women occupy a place in many ways distinct from those of men. In general they are hired for jobs of material and emotional upkeep of persons and/or for subordinate jobs in various work processes. The ill-paying, little valued, non-union jobs are their lot. They are the reserve labor cushion whose fate depends on the fluctuations of the economy.
>
> (Juteau and Laurin, 1989, p. 30)

Similarly, Grant (1995) points out that, during World War II, the war economy and the departure of men for military service drastically altered the pattern of public-sector employment for women. Before the war, paid employment outside the home was a necessity for poor women, but for more affluent women paid employment was seen to be as incompatible with marriage. These women might work in such traditional women's jobs as teaching, nursing or social work, but only until marriage. During the war, the demand for an unskilled, low-paid non-union work-force was met by women. In the UK, all women between the ages of 18 and 45 years were required to register for employment, and women who had been barred from jobs outside the home now found themselves employable. While women acquired new confidence in their abilities to participate in the paid work-force, when the war ended the majority of them returned home in order to vacate their jobs for the returning soldiers. Thus market need rather than women's choice determined their access to paid employment.

Similarly, Juteau and Laurin's (1989) study of Quebecoise nuns shows that, until the 1960s, the nuns were the main providers of Quebec's health, education and social services. When the state assumed exclusive responsibility for these services, the nuns were replaced by lay women workers who undertook paid employment. The entry of these women into the work-force marginalized the nuns and led to their eventual disappearance from the service sector. At the same time, as in the British example given above, paid employment was perceived as being incompatible with marriage, so the lay professional woman either gave up work for marriage or marriage for work. Thus again women's options with regard to paid employment were not under their control.

In this context, the ideology of altruism becomes a powerful mechanism of social and economic control over those who perform service work. In order to promote the image of nursing in the USA in the early part of this century, nursing leaders promoted the ideals of altruism and service. This contributes to the economic devaluation of nursing labour, and its susceptibility to market forces. Turkoski writes that:

> Altruism and service become a form of self-coercion that makes economic inequality and asymmetry appear normal, natural and desirable as the badge of professional status.
>
> (Turkoski, 1992, p. 157)

Thus in the shift from private duty to hospital nursing which took place when private individuals could no longer afford to hire nursing services during the Great Depression, and as the federal government began to support the development of hospitals and the health-care industry, nursing leaders persuaded the nursing rank and file to accept wages and working conditions from hospitals which were not economically too exacting. Instead, the ideals of vocation and service attracted women into socially acceptable nursing work (Turkoski, 1992).

In the USA, a brief shortage of nurses in the 1980s led to substantial wage increases, but this job market favouring nurses was short-lived. As health-care costs soared, schemes were introduced to contain them. The federal government instituted a prospective payment system for Medicare and Medicaid, which subsidize health care for the elderly and indigent. Under prospective payment, hospitals are paid a fixed fee for diagnostic related categories (DRGs), rather than for actual patient costs or length of hospital stay. Private insurance companies followed suit, negotiating reimbursement rates with hospitals.

Nurses have been among the first casualties of these economic stringencies. As a group, they are expensive, accounting for half the work-force and a quarter of the NHS budget (Buchan, 1992). In the USA, nurses account for 28 per cent of total hospital costs (Gordon, 1995). Under cost constraints, US employers attempt to reduce the costs of nursing labour by making each nurse carry a greater workload, taking on additional duties and additional patients (Gordon, 1991b), and/or by replacing registered nurses with cheaper, less skilled personnel (Gray, 1993; Scott, 1993). In the UK, many nursing skills are seen by managers and policy makers as 'unspecialized, interchangeable and therefore easily transferable' (James, 1991, cited in Hart, 1991).

In an analysis of a nursing strike in the USA, Levi (1980) attributes the vulnerability of the nursing profession to its 'functional redundancy': other personnel can take on many of the tasks that nurses perform, and nurses can take on many of the tasks performed by others. Thus less skilled ancillary personnel dispose of refuse, answer phones, stock supplies, feed and bath patients, yet nurses can (and do) take on all of these tasks in addition to skilled nursing. At the same time, nurses can perform many of the tasks done by respiratory therapists, physical therapists and junior doctors. Thus the boundaries of nursing practice are neither firmly set, nor fully under the control of those who practise nursing. Within certain legal limits, the work that nurses do can be expanded or reduced to suit the labour needs of the employer.

It has been possible for nurses to take advantage of the change in market forces. For example, in the USA, the Denver Nursing Project which cares for people with HIV/AIDS has been able to respond creatively to the apparently negative changes associated with health-care reforms. They have been able to curb costs by using their skills to replace physicians' more expensive and often less appropriate skills (Schroeder, 1993). The project has been funded by a federal grant and three local hospitals. This nurse-led service in partnership with clients provides an alternative to hospital treatment, and saved an estimated million dollars in 1992. Savings are derived from the lower costs of out-patient treatment, and from the formation of effective, stable nurse–client partnerships. Nursing skills have reduced costs and made a qualitative difference in patients' lives.

Similarly, in a review of advanced practice nursing in the USA, Safriet (1992) relates the development of the role to the search to contain costs in the US health-care market. Safriet makes a number of points concerning both the quality and the cost-effectiveness of the advanced practice nurse (APN) compared with the physician. First, the APN improves client access to health care, particularly among low-income groups in inner city and rural areas that are less popular with physicians. Secondly, training costs are lower for APNs than for physicians. Thirdly, the APN's scope of practice is wider than the physician's, encompassing preventive, counselling and diagnostic activities. Fourthly, on average APNs spend more time with fewer clients than physicians, because they combine both medical and nursing activities within their consultation. Finally, patients who choose to see an APN appear to be more satisfied with their care than those who choose an equivalent consultation with a physician.

The move towards advanced practice roles, while encouraged in both the USA and the UK as part of health-care reforms, may offer nurses new challenges but also expose their vulnerability to market forces. By developing alternative models of professional caring practice, they may find themselves being used as cost-cutting devices and cheaper alternatives to physicians. The caring aspects of the job may remain unrecognized as nurses develop ways of giving quality care at lower costs than medically dominated or delivered services.

However, Safriet believes that there are ways of preventing the APN from being seen as a cheaper alternative to physicians, and advocates the same rate of payment for the same job. While recognizing that this argument may run counter to a health service determined to cut costs, she is of the opinion that APNs' overall costs would still be less than those of physicians because of their less expensive treatment preferences.

In the UK, Hart (1991) describes a less optimistic situation in which the 'managerial-medical' model of health care may mean that the 'nursing skills are devalued and down-graded, or up-graded and valued only to the extent that nurses take over the low status and routine technical work of junior doctors'. She sees this model as an attractive one for managers who need to cut their unit costs in order to compete in the emerging health-care market.

Evidence from the UK suggests that the implementation of the market, the breakup of the National Health Service into semi-autonomous Trusts, and the purchaser/provider divide have indeed driven a rift between those who give care and those who are responsible for managing its organization and finance.[9,10] A study of morale among community nurses and health visitors in three first-wave English Trusts during the first 3 years of health-care reforms revealed that front-line staff experienced a conflict of values between finance-oriented managers and their own commitment to care. The following quote represents a prevailing view among nurses in this study: 'Money has replaced the patient in our focus of care. We need to resist this insidious erosion to our commitment to people' (Traynor and Wade, 1994, p. 43).

On the other hand, managers in this study were found to believe that a 'business ethos' was highly compatible with the principles of good health care. Surveys in the USA revealed similar findings, with many changes being made in hospitals by administrators with a 'we know best' attitude who did not value 'hands on care' (Noble 1993).

A significant effect of the market on nursing in the UK is to attempt to reduce operating costs by reducing nurses' pay. Formerly paid according to a national pay scale, nurses now see their pay as being set by Trusts that are in competition with each other. Their angry reaction to the government's 1994 one per cent pay deal is evidence of their growing awareness of the negative effects of the market on health care in general and nursing in particular. They are even contemplating industrial action supported by a range of organizations, including the Royal College of Nursing – which has until now been opposed to such measures. The introduction of the internal market is being blamed for increased workloads, particularly paperwork, and threats to quality of patient care. In short, nurses feel that they are being expected to do more for less.

It is interesting to see the language of the market being adopted by the Royal College of Nursing in support of their members when they state that:

> If Trusts lose their qualified nurses, they cannot hope to compete for health
> service contracts in a competitive market. If a neighbouring Trust is prepared to

meet the award in full, or even to pay more than 3 per cent, increasing numbers will simply vote with their feet.

(Royal College of Nursing, 1995).

Whether Trust managers, like governments and private health-care corporations, are concerned about retaining qualified nurses or paying them adequately depends on whether they regard them as having unique rather than interchangeable skills. One approach to convincing them that the former is the case is to accumulate evidence that skilled nursing matters.

Value of skilled nursing

Some preliminary attempts have been made to verify the value of skilled nursing care.

In the UK in 1991, the Audit Commission, the public finance watchdog, reported that one of the biggest problems facing health care in the UK was the 'undervaluing of nursing and nurses', which in turn prevented the efficient use of ward nursing resources (Audit Commission, 1991).

● A US survey has revealed that three out of five nurses believed that cost containment had a detrimental effect on quality of care in their hospitals (Collins, 1988). Nearly 75 per cent of respondents felt that cost containment left 'no time for a caring attitude'. The little things, defined as 'psychological support, teaching, frequent turning and positioning' were the first items to go because nurses felt pressured to perform the visible 'high-tech' routines. The false economy of reducing skilled nursing is illustrated by the example of pressure sores, which may develop as a result of inadequate nursing care and which cost more to treat than to prevent (McSweeney, 1994). A federally funded study further confirmed the negative effect of cost containment on quality of care, suggesting higher death rates in hospitals facing stiff competition and stringent state regulation (cited in Collins, 1988).

A reduction in the number of skilled nursing staff appears to be a major reason for this situation, because fewer registered nurses means managing crises rather than planning care. For example, early in 1993 the *New York Times* article cited above also reported the findings of a survey which revealed that, although wages had risen, so had workloads. As a result, nurses were exhausted and patient care was undermined (Noble, 1993).

There is growing evidence for a direct correlation between qualified staff, good standards of care and positive patient outcomes (Scott, 1993).

But as a leading US nurse states:

> The value of nursing derives from the content of its work. Nurses care for those who cannot care for themselves; such compassion is a hallmark of a civilized society. . . . Whether this care is supplied through the public sector or, as is much more common, through the private sector, there is a consensus that care should be given when it is needed. But we hate to pay for it.

(Lynaugh, 1988, p. VII-2)

We return full circle to the question which we posed at the beginning of this chapter, namely how to get at this complex phenomenon called care in order to make it visible and valued in a market-oriented society committed to costs. In the final section of this chapter we shall consider to what extent critical research methodologies can contribute to the study of care and its context.

Towards a critical understanding of care

In this chapter we have discussed the attitudes and activities of care and their association with nursing work. To an understanding of nursing work drawn from the nursing literature we have added an understanding of nursing labour. We have found that nurses are the principal professional providers of health care in both the public and the private health-care sectors, yet nursing labour is characterized by gender division, subordination, marginalization in public awareness and policy, and vulnerability to market forces.

Our critical understanding of care draws on critical theory, but goes beyond critical theory to draw on feminist theory as well.[9,11]

Many studies of nurses take a phenomenological perspective. We find this perspective limited because it emphasizes individual experiences and interpretations. Critical theory demands that we situate phenomena within their historical and social context, and it asks not only what is happening, but why, and whose interests are being served.

In order to answer the questions raised by critical theory, we need to draw on feminist theory as well. Combining these perspectives we can see that it is no accident that care-givers are women and that care work is under-recognized and undervalued. Present-day nursing-care arrangements reflect underlying social, political and economic assumptions about the nature and value of women's caring work. The profession of nursing is a women's profession, built on assumptions about women's natural skills in nurturing and their innate orientation towards care. Historically, it reflects values imported from the domestic sphere as the nursing profession emerged during the Victorian era (Levi 1980; Hughes, 1990).

In its professionalization project, nursing has faced two major challenges. The first is to carve out an area of practice in which professional nursing is distinct from medicine and from non-professional or lay care-giving. The second is to establish and hold a position within a health-care delivery system that is dominated primarily by medicine and increasingly by health-care administration.

In carving out an area of practice, nursing has laid claim to a distinctive combination of attitude and skill. This commitment to care and expertise in care-giving is indeed a distinctive feature of nursing practice. However, the skills and effort involved in caring work are too easily obscured by the image of calling or vocation. The commitment of nurses to care is claimed as a practical and moral imperative and as a moral covenant (Bishop and Scudder, 1990). This moral language builds a self-image and public image of nurses as selfless and devoted, motivated by vocation and feeling rather than by material concerns, but it does not serve the profession well in holding its position within the health-care system.

Nursing has adopted the language and ethos of care without sufficient critical examination of where this ethos comes from and whose interests it represents. In nursing, the ethos of care contributes heavily to the gender division of labour and the subordination of nurses. When nurses present themselves as uniquely committed to care, it is very difficult for them to argue about the terms and conditions under which they perform their caring work and sell their caring labour. Nursing strikes are problematic not only because others can step in and perform the tasks which nurses perform, but also because the withdrawal of nursing services undercuts the very professional image which nursing has built up (Levi, 1980).

Condon (1992) suggests that caring provides a new and authentic metaphor for nursing, grounded in women's direct experience as mothers, nurses and care-givers. Freely chosen, the metaphor of care can point the way to a personal and social ethic; nursing is a 'space' in which this can happen. From the perspective of critical theory, however, nursing cannot establish a space unconnected with the values and structures of society. Even if the nurse chooses this space and his or her activities within it, the space itself and his or her choices and actions are shaped by the external context. In our view, we cannot understand nursing fully without understanding how attitudes, behaviours and opportunities in our society are shaped by gender, and how they operate in all spheres to diminish the economic value placed on women's work.

Feminist theory brings us to the paradox of care (Gordon, 1991a) – can we continue to value care without perpetuating the structures of subordination and exploitation within which the work and labour of care have traditionally been situated? According to Gordon, some feminists say that this cannot be done, and therefore measure women's progress by how far and how effectively we are able to distance ourselves from care-giving. However, we share with Gordon the hope that we can 'keep the market-place in its place' and organize care-giving in ways that reaffirm this basic human capacity.

Conclusions

Even as we attempt to define it, the role of the nurse in health-care delivery is changing drastically. We are in danger of recognizing the contributions of nurses only by losing them, encapsulated in the words of the popular song, 'you don't know what you've got till it's gone'.[9,12] Our attempts to define what nurses do, and to account for how nursing work is appropriated as nursing labour, acquire particular urgency.

Our present arrangements are the result of a particular social and economic history in which professional nurses have made and continue to make significant contributions to health care. We should be cautious about abandoning these arrangements and replacing them with others before we have a clear idea of what we are giving up and what we are gaining or losing.

Central to our discussion is our concern with both individual and social responses to the human need for care. We suggest that neither the work of care-giving nor the moral commitment to care can be abandoned, but that we must examine critically the social arrangements which determine who provides care and the terms and conditions under which they do so. Far more than individual vocation or moral commitment, these social arrangements inhibit or sustain our capacity to care.

Endnotes

9.1.   Exceptions include:

Ashley JA (1976) *Hospitals, Paternalism and the Role of the Nurse.* Teachers College Press, New York.

Glazer N (1993) *Women's Paid and Unpaid Labor.* Temple University Press, Philadelphia.

Melosh B (1982) *The Physician's Hand: Work and Conflict in American Nursing.* Temple University Press, Philadelphia.

Reverby S (1987) *Ordered to Care: the Dilemma of American Nursing 1850–1945.* Cambridge University Press, Cambridge.

Strauss A *et al.* (1985) *Social Organization of Medical Work.* University of Chicago Press, Chicago.

For further discussion, see Carpenter M (1993) The subordination of nurses in health care: towards a social divisions approach. In Riska E and Wegar K (eds) *Gender, Work and Medicine.* Sage, London. Carpenter points out the historical neglect of nursing in sociological research, acknowledges recent efforts to correct this, and warns against a 'ghettoized' sociology of nursing, marginalized from the main discipline of sociology in the way that nursing is marginalized in health care.

9.2.   Oakley A (1986) On the importance of being a nurse. In *Telling the Truth about Jerusalem: A Collection of Essays and Poems.* Basil Blackwell, New York.

9.3.   For a typology of medical work which includes comfort work and sentimental work, see Strauss *et al.* (1985).

9.4.   Levi (1980, p. 336) refers to the 'functional redundancy' of nursing: nursing has developed in such a way that substitutions for what nurses do can be made from both above and below; thus nursing cannot maintain a firm hold on its own scope of practice and professional territory.

9.5.   See Smith (1992, pp. 197–8). This term from the feminist literature refers to predominant trends in Western thought, recently challenged by feminists, which perceive the world in dualistic terms: mind/body, objective/subjective, and abstract/concrete.

9.6.   Midwifery is a particularly stark example of medical domination of a women's occupational group. US privatized health care ensures that obstetrics is a particularly lucrative specialty. Until recently, obstetricians successfully opposed nurse-midwives delivering babies and limited their conditions of practice. Now, the increasing number of lay midwives, who rely on acquiring knowledge and skills through apprenticeships and resist any form of medicalization, are facing prosecutions and arrests instigated by the medical establishment. One report bluntly states that 'where neighbourhoods sport an obstetrician on every sunny block, the climate is hostile to midwives' (Ohland, 1993). In other words, obstetricians oppose midwives setting up practices in the same neighbourhoods because they see them as competition, as they offer cheaper alternatives to obstetric care. In the UK, midwives have been able to practise independently since the 1902 Midwives' Act. Obstetricians, however, have still been able to use their professional dominance and power to regulate and control pregnancy and childbirth. Over the years, the shift in the number of births taking place in hospitals rather than womens' own homes with only midwives in attendance and the growth of sophisticated technological interventions, are testimonies to the obstetricians' success.

9.7.   We refer here to the notion of patriarchy as stated by Rosaldo and Lamphere (1974) and cited by Dahlerup: 'Everywhere we find that women are excluded from certain economic or political activities, that their roles as wives and mothers are associated with fewer powers and prerogatives than are the roles of men. It seems fair to say, then, that all contemporary societies are to some extent male dominated, and although the degree and expression of female subordination vary greatly, sexual asymmetry is presently a universal fact of human life (Dahlerup, 1987, p. 3).' Dahlerup (1987) notes that common to all definitions of patriarchy is the focus on men's power, authority or dominance over women, particularly over women's sexuality and labour.

9.8.   Shue (1980) makes a useful distinction between systemic oppression, in which arrangements that exploit some members of society to the advantage of others are built into the structure of society and widely taken for granted, and systematic oppression, in which deliberate attempts are made, through legislation, segregation or coercive force, to oppress individuals or groups.

9.9.   For an excellent discussion of the limitations of the public/private split, see Juteau and Laurin (1989). In a rigorous review of the feminist literature, and a specific study of Quebecoise nuns, Juteau and Laurin argue that (1) gender relations function as do class relations, to equate the interests of the dominant group(s) with the collective or general interest, and (2) this results in both private and collective appropriation of women's labour in 'a diversity of sites, places, relations and institutions'.

9.10. Although the factors contributing to cost containment and competition in the US health-care market differ from those in the UK, the effects are similar (Smith, 1996).

9.11. See Campbell and Bunting (1991). Critical theory integrates subjective perceptions, interpretations and belief systems with Marxist political-economic analysis to provide a richer account of social phenomena than is provided by either crude Marxism or phenomenology. Feminist theory provides key insights into particular features of women's social position and experiences.

9.12.   Joni Mitchell (1969) 'Big Yellow Taxi', from the record album *Ladies of the Canyon*, Burbank, Warner Brothers Record Company and New York, Siquomb Publishing Company.

References

Ashley JA (1976) *Hospitals, Paternalism and the Role of the Nurse*. Teachers College Press, New York.
Audit Commission (1991) *The Virtue of Patients*. HMSO, London.
Baxter C (1988) *The Black Nurse: An Endangered Species*. Cambridge National Extension College for Training in Health and Race, Cambridge.
Beardshaw V and Robinson R (1990) *New for Old? Prospects for Nursing in the 1990s*. King's Fund Institute, London.
Benner P and Wrubel J (1989) *The Primacy of Caring*. Addison-Wesley, Menlo Park, CA.
Bishop A and Scudder J (1990) *The Practical, Moral, and Personal Sense of Nursing*. State University Press of New York, Albany, NY.
Buchan J (1992) *Flexibility or Fragmentation? Trends and Prospects in Nurse Pay*. King's Fund Institute, London.
Campbell J and Bunting S (1991) Voices and paradigms: perspectives on critical and feminist theory in nursing. *Advances in Nursing Science* 13, 1–15.
Carpenter M (1993) The subordination of nurses in health care: towards a social divisions approach. In Riska E and Wegar K (eds) *Gender, Work and Medicine* pp. 95–130. Sage, London.
Collins HL (1988) When the profit motive threatens patient care. *Registered Nurse* 10, 8, 74–83.
Condon EH (1992) Nursing and the caring metaphor: gender and political influences on an ethics of care. *Nursing Outlook* 40, 14–19.
Dahlerup D (1987) Confusing concepts – confusing reality: a theoretical discussion of the patriarchal state in Showstack. In Sassoon A Showstach (ed.) *Women and the State*, pp. 93–127. Routledge, London.
Finch J and Groves D (1983) *A Labour of Love: Women, Work and Caring*. Routledge & Kegan Paul, London.
Freidson E (1970) *Profession of Medicine: A Study of the Sociology of Applied Knowledge*. Dodd Mead, New York.
Freund PES and McGuire MB (1991) *Health, Illness and the Social Body: A Critical Sociology*. Prentice Hall, Englewood Cliffs.
Gaze H (1987) Man appeal: men in nursing. *Nursing Times* 83, 20, 24–9.
Glazer N (1993) *Women's Paid and Unpaid Labor*. Temple University Press, Philadelphia.
Gordon S (1991a) Fear of caring: the feminist paradox. *American Journal of Nursing* 91, 48.
Gordon S (1991b) *Prisoners of Men's Dreams*, Little, Brown and Co., Boston.
Gordon S (1995) Is there a nurse in the house? *The Nation*, 13 February, p. 199.
Grant L (1995) Keep smiling through. *The Guardian Society* 3 May, pp. 5–6.
Gray B (1993) RN job market shifts as health system evolves. *Nurse Week* 6, 24, 1–23.
Hart E (1991) Ghost in the machine. *Health Services Journal* 101, 20–2.
Hartmann H (1979) Capitalism, patriarchy and job segregation. In Einstein Z (ed.)

Capitalism, Patriarchy and the Case for Socialist Feminism. Monthly Review Press, New York.

Hochschild AR (1983) *The Managed Heart: Commercialization of Human Feeling.* University of California Press, Berkeley, CA.

Hochschild AR (1989) *The Second Shift – Working Parents and the Revolution at Home.* Viking/UK Piatkus Press, New York.

Hughes L (1990) Professionalizing domesticity: a synthesis of selected nursing historiography. *Advances in Nursing Science* 12, 25–31.

James V (1991) *Changing Babies.*Unpublished Report, Department of Nursing Studies, Nottingham University.

Juteau D and Laurin N (1989) From nuns to surrogate mothers: evolution of the forms of the appropriation of women. *Feminist Issues* 9, 13–40.

Kramer M and Schmalenberg C (1988) Magnet hospitals: Part I. Institutions of excellence. *Journal of Nursing Administration* 18, 13–24.

Leininger M (1990) Historic and epistemologic dimensions of care and caring with future directions. In Stevenson J and Tripp-Reimer T (eds) *Knowledge About Care and Caring*, pp. 19–31. American Academy of Nursing, Kansas City.

Levi M (1980) Functional redundancy and the process of professionalization: the case of registered nurses in the United States. *Journal of Health Policy, Politics and Law* 5, 333–53.

Lynaugh J (1988) *Twice as Many and Still Not Enough.* US Commission on Nursing, US Department of Health and Human Services, Washington.

McIntosh M (1978) The state and the oppression of women. In Kuhn A and Wolpe AM (eds) *Feminism and Materialism*, pp. 254–89. Routledge, London.

McSweeney P (1994) Assessing the cost of pressure sores. *Nursing Standard* 8, 25–6.

Noble BP (1993) Pushing nurses to a breaking point. *New York Times*, 10 January.

Noddings N (1984) *Caring: A Feminine Approach to Ethics and Moral Education.* University of California Press, Berkeley, CA.

Oakley A (1984) The importance of being a nurse. *Nursing Times* 80, 24–7.

Oakley A (1986) On the importance of being a nurse. In *Telling the Truth about Jerusalem: A Collection of Essays and Poems*. Basil Blackwell, New York.

Ohland G (1993) Birthing at gunpoint. *San Francisco Weekly*, 18 August, p. 7.

Ray MA (1987) Technological caring: a new model in critical care. *Dimensions of Critical Care in Nursing* 6, 166–73.

Renzetti C and Lee R (1992) *Researching Sensitive Topics.* Sage, London.

Reverby S (1987) *Ordered to Care.* Cambridge University Press, Cambridge.

Riska E (1993) Introduction. In Riska E and Wegar K (eds) *Gender, Work and Medicine*, pp. 1–12. Sage, London.

Robinson K (1992) The nursing workforce: aspects of inequality. In Robinson J, Gray A and Elkan R (eds) *Policy Issues in Nursing*, pp. 24–37. Open University Press, Milton Keynes.

Rosaldo MZ and Lamphere L (1974) *Women, Culture and Society.* Stanford University Press, Stanford.

Royal College of Nursing (1995) *3% Now – Fair Deal for Nurses. Campaign Leaflet, No. 000 512.* Royal College of Nursing, London.

Safriet BJ (1992) Health care dollars and regulatory sense: the role of advanced practice nursing (especially nurse practitioners and certified nurse midwives). *Yale Journal on Regulation* 6, 417–88.

Salvage J (1985) *The Politics of Nursing.* Heinemann, London.

Schroeder C (1993) Nursing's response to the crisis of access, costs and quality in health care. *Advances in Nursing Science* 16, 1–20.

Scott K (1993) RN layoffs of growing concern to ANA. *The American Nurse* 25, 3, 14.

Shue H (1980) *Basic Rights.* Princeton University Press, Princeton, NJ.

Smith P (1992) *The Emotional Labour of Nursing.* Macmillan Press, Basingstoke.

Smith P (1996) Health care reform in Britain and the United States – Public or market-led? – a review. *International Journal of Public Administration*, in press.

Strauss A, Fagerhaugh S, Suczek B and Weiner C (1985) *Social Organization of Medical Work.* University of Chicago Press, Chicago.

Traynor M and Wade B (1994) *The Morale of Nurses Working in the Community: A Study of Three NHS Trusts: Year 3.* The Daphne Heald Research Unit, Royal College of Nursing, London.

Turkoski BB (1992) A critical analysis of professionalism in nursing. In Thompson JL, Allen DG and Rodrigues-Fisher L (eds) *Critique, Resistance and Action: Working Papers on the Politics of Nursing*, pp. 149–65. National League for Nursing, New York.

Ungerson C (1983) Why do women care? In Finch J and Groves D (eds) *A Labour of Love: Women, Work and Caring*, pp. 31–49. Routledge & Kegan Paul, London.

Waerness K (1987) On the rationality of caring. In Showsack Sasson A (ed.) *Women and the State*, pp. 207–34. Routledge, London.

Ward D (1993) The kin care trap: the unpaid labor of long-term care. *Socialist Review* 23, 83–105.

Witz A (1992) *Professions and Patriarchy.* Routledge, London.

Further reading

Savage J (1995) *Nursing Intimacy: An Ethnographic Approach to Nurse–Patient Interaction.* Scutari Press, London.

Smith P (1992) *The Emotional Labour of Nursing.* Macmillan Press, Basingstoke.

Index

Scholars whose ideas are discussed appear in the index by name only as complete references follow each chapter.